free TO HEAL

Advance Praise

"Got it! Reading & can't stop… I have to say you are an inspiration!"
—**Jane Porter-Green**

"I devoured this book in 3 days! I cried at the beginning because all I saw was my story too. I'm not a medical doctor but was in a soul sucking waitress job with what seemed like no way out. Dr. Shaunna's story resonates with me and her steps to creating a successful Health Coaching practice are so clear and precise."
—**Linda Rietmann**, Certified Health Coach, Balance Health Coaching, NJ

"What I loved best about this book is it is very easy to understand! Dr. Shaunna's heart is in the book spoken from Love. This book is 'off the charts' beneficial for health coaches. A must have! The tools in this book are priceless. My favourite tool is seriously, the elevator. I have already attracted, and I am coaching my ideal clients following the steps in this book! *Free to Heal* is a must read for anyone wanting to find the secret of success."
—**Rachel Borntrager**, Certified Health Coach, Gut Health Coach, Whole and Well Co.

"This book is the single most effective tool you need as a health coach. Stop dreaming about starting your business and use the tools and game plan to start living your soul-satisfying dream today!"
—**Debra Moss**, Certified Health Coach

"Motivational! Inspirational! Transformational! Thank you Dr. Shaunna for your knowledge and guidance with this long-awaited book for anyone seeking to build a career as a Health Coach. Your contagious spirit and soul have uplifted me in many ways. Feeling blessed."

—**Aimee Hyatt**, Health Coach, Founder of DogaFit

"Dr. Shaunna provides guidance that is insightful, thoughtful and real. It's obvious that she truly wants coaches to succeed in healing themselves and their clients. She makes a seemingly unreachable goal approachable and feasible. In addition to a tremendous amount of hope, she includes practical steps and potential pitfalls. Her guidance is helping me on my own journey of reclaiming my purpose and my life!"

—**Dr. Selvi Vasudevan**, Medical Doctor, Certified Health Coach

"I was struggling to launch as a Health Coach—Not anymore! This is not a read once book. This is a Manual. Dr Shaunna gives a practical step by step process not only to build a successful health business but also a successful life. Forever indebted for the wisdom shared."

—**Lana Kirtley**, Certified Health Coach,
Empowering Health Journeys

"*Free to Heal* has excellent, clear steps for health coaches to be all and more for clients with communication skills for success. A real Awakened Healer story! We all need to prevent the chronic diseases that can be avoided. This informative book shows us how we have more control than we realize with our own health. Meditation is good for the soul! Thank you Dr. Shaunna Menard for lighting our way!"

—**Patricia Pottinger**

"If learning how to find a niche that truly resonates with you was all you got out of this book, it would be worth its weight in gold! Total. Game. Changer."

—**Jennifer Bago** Health Coach Ltd, Specializing in Women's Reproductive Health

"Dr Shaunna has done all the heavy lifting! Her 9 (simple/easy to understand) steps and ample words of wisdom cut a clear path through thousands of dollars in expense, countless hours of trial and error, through the underbrush of the entrepreneurial jungle so that we, aspiring and passionate health coaches, can avoid the pitfalls she so successfully navigated and get to what we can do best while fulfilling our soul's purpose…heal!

—**Marianne Koszorus**, Certified Health Coach, Live360Wellness

"As healers it often seems that if we want our career, the prevailing system compromises our health, whereas if we prioritise wellbeing with an awakened lifestyle, we risk our finances. This book helps the reader to discover the bridge between the two with an awakening that it is possible without our worst fears coming true, but instead finding satisfaction through practical measures to reach our dreams."

—**Elizabeth Plant**, Massage Therapist & Health Coach, UK

"I am so thankful I heard Dr. Shaunna speak at IIN National Conference and that I am in her Awakened Healers group and have her book as a permanent guide! Coming from a medical background, the entrepreneurial process seems insurmountable. Her mentorship, positive enthusiasm, easy to relate to steps, and encouragement are a

Godsend! Looking forward to a great new career into my retirement from ICU nursing."

—**Donna Rae**, Certified Health Coach, RN Patient Advocate,
Passages 2 Health

"*Free to Heal* and the Awakened Healer process is a life changing gift to the health coaching community. Following the steps in the book and being a part of the signature program, I was able to visualize my perfect client and put together the steps for my program. I am honored to have been part of this process and to be featured in the introduction. That conversation sealed my commitment to my passion of helping Dads across the world with blood sugar issues."

—**Tim Pedersen**, Integrative Health and Nutrition Coach, Dad
Bod Warrior

"*Free to Heal* is an easy, fun read written with truth and love. This book is a combination of passion and love. After reading this book, I feel empowered to keep coaching and sharing nutritional dense super foods."

—**Nic Uyeno**

"Loved the style and substance of the book. I am not a healer but truly believe healing oneself is the first step. An easy read that makes you ponder at some points and just keep reading at others. So well done Shaunna. Thank you!"

—**Lorna Ved**

"At first glance this book seems to be primarily for Health Care Professionals, Life Coaches, Holistic Entrepreneur's, Healing

Coaches etc. Wait! Keep reading the book even if you are not one of the mentioned. In one way or another we are all helpers and healers. I have always led my life wanting to help others. This book is for everyone. Even if the only person you help, heal or coach is yourself. YOU WIN as does everyone around you!!… This is a fantastic read for all!"

—**Joann Smiley**

free TO HEAL

9 STEPS
to a Successful,
Soul-Satisfying
Health Coaching
Practice

SHAUNNA MENARD, MD

NEW YORK

LONDON • NASHVILLE • MELBOURNE • VANCOUVER

Table of Contents

Foreword

It is no secret that there is a global health care crisis today. Rates of chronic disease continue to rise as trillions of dollars are spent every year in the U.S. alone. People are going through life at hyper speed— not feeding their bodies nutritious foods, not sleeping well and not moving their bodies nearly enough. Most doctors' visits are for stress-related complaints. Chronic diseases are now the leading cause of death and disability in the U.S. and growing globally and lifestyle factors such as diet, exercise, sleep, and stress are a huge determinant. But every day I hear amazing stories of transformation that reinforce my belief that people can make simple changes that can dramatically improve their health. However, people often need help to make these simple changes that create these life-changing results.

When I started the Institute for Integrative Nutrition (IIN) in 1992, I was just one person with a simple idea that if I could change what people ate, I could change the world. I didn't want to just create a school. I wanted to create a healthy movement. Our mission at

IIN is "to play a crucial role in improving health and happiness and through that process, create a ripple effect that transforms the world." Since its inception, IIN has evolved from live classes in New York to now an innovative online learning platform, that has trained over 100,000 health coaches in over 150 countries.

The role of health coaches is becoming increasingly critical. Traditional doctors and other health professionals are on the frontlines of helping those in need, but they don't always have the time or resources to help patients build healthy habits. In addition, our food supply has become increasingly complex—artificial even. People are seriously challenged navigating confusing food labels and contradictory nutritional theories and trying to fit 'one size fits all' recommendations. Are eggs a good source of protein or a bad source of cholesterol? Does milk do a body good or not? Does an office worker require the same diet as someone who does physical labor? A November 2015 study published in *Cell* found that universal recommendations simply don't work. Researchers gathered data on blood sugar response from 800 people and 46,000 meals and found that each person had a different response to similar foods. Studying and working in the field of nutrition for over thirty years, bio-individuality is something I've always known to be true. So how can we have customized health care at this level? And what about what I call 'primary foods'—things like relationships, activity, career, and spirituality? A person stuck in an unhealthy relationship can eat all the broccoli in the world, but it won't change that relationship which will cause their health and well-being to suffer. The energy spent at a draining job will also negatively impact health and outweigh the benefits of just eating healthy. So how can we truly address our global health crisis at this personal level?

We have a demand for a new kind of health advocate that fills a significant and growing void in our current healthcare system. Health coaches are the perfect solution to fill the void and bridge the gap between doctors and their patients. Health coaches work with clients to make the necessary shifts from unhealthy habits to sustainable, healthy ones. As more doctors have begun to see the value of nutrition, movement, and other lifestyle factors, more of them have begun to work with health coaches in their practice to serve their patients better. Health coaches can help patients stay accountable to their doctor's recommendations and customize them to their particular circumstances. It is one thing to recommend someone lose weight. A health coach, however, can address the nutritional nuances of a particular person, their emotional eating and stressful lifestyle and give them the guidance, ongoing support, resources and coaching to allow the patient to be successful in carrying out that recommendation.

IIN health coaches have made tremendous strides in improving global wellness over the past twenty-five years. They have raised awareness that food changes everything and highlighted the food/mood connection and that we truly are what we eat. Our graduates have helped thousands of people throughout the world transform their health, prevent disease, and live more balanced lives. They have played a role in school food programs, educating the public through television and other media and influencing government policy. One of our "superstar graduates" is Dr. Shaunna Menard who has done all of the aforementioned. She has been a huge inspiration and supporter of health coaches and the critical role these pioneers play in health care. She has spoken on numerous occasions to our students and graduates as a visiting IIN teacher.

As a medical doctor, Dr. Shaunna experienced first-hand that people had more power to impact their health than they realized but they weren't exercising this power. She knew that if she could reach people earlier and help educate and coach them to better lifestyle choices that this could prevent needless suffering. This is what inspired her to become a student herself at IIN a decade ago attending live classes in New York which is where I first met her. In 2018, when she was the emcee of our annual conference, it was evident that there was a small but growing number of doctors now in the audience—a positive trend that had occurred over the past decade with more health professionals wanting to know how they could best support their patients. The ripple effect has continued to grow. As more and more graduates have desired to make health coaching their life's work, it is invaluable to take direction from someone who has already carved out that path and built a thriving practice. Dr. Shaunna's journey to break *Free to Heal*, will undoubtedly prove inspirational, instructional and empowering for both new and seasoned health coaches, and other health professionals. There are many important factors to consider if health coaches desire to transition to a successful, health coaching practice as their livelihood. Dr. Shaunna clearly outlines this process with an easy to follow and comprehensive, step-by-step approach to become a successful, holistic entrepreneur.

Free to Heal is a delightful and powerful read that is written with all of the passion, heart, lightness, and leadership that is characteristic of Dr. Shaunna. I know she has used the principles she shares in this book with her father and her own health coaching clients. Everyone, including those who don't yet see themselves as healers, will appreciate the lessons in this book for their own health and healing. It is a pleasure to collaborate with a like-minded health professional committed to improving health and happiness and being a part of the ripple effect that is transforming the world.

— **Joshua Rosenthal**, MScEd, Founder of Institute
for Integrative Nutrition, New York

Introduction

"The doctor of the future will give no medicine, but will interest his patient in the care of the human frame, in diet and in the cause and prevention of disease."
–Thomas Edison

Dear loving healer, read on. The life you save may just be your own.

"The difference you can make is massive! The world needs you now more than ever. The work you are doing is so important!" said Alex, one of my clients who was also a nurse on the vascular surgery floor. She was speaking to another client of mine, certified health coach Tim, who was creating his signature program to help diabetic dads lose weight and balance their blood sugars. Alex told our Awakened Healers group that there were a lot of amputations on the vascular surgery ward where she worked—and a lot of them are diabetic. "One man, a father in his early fifties, just had double above knee amputations from diabetes. This is really ruining his life. He has been in hospital for 370 days. One amputation became infected and then the other. It is a real nightmare." (500 amputations are performed every day in America and seventy-five percent are related to diabetes. Forty to eighty percent will die within five years of their diabetic amputation.)

It doesn't have to be this way! Sixty percent of Americans now have at least one chronic disease like diabetes, heart disease, stroke, or cancer, and these are among the leading causes of death and the leading causes of health care costs. The World Health Organization states that eighty percent of all heart disease, stroke, and type 2 diabetes and forty percent of cancers can be prevented. So, if these deadly and costly chronic diseases can be prevented, why aren't they? Why are the rates of all chronic disease on the rise? How and who can stop this crazy thing?

The other side of the equation are these amazing people who feel called to help and heal. Doctors, nurses, technologists, and other allied health professionals began their careers full of hope and promise to make this world a healthier, happier place. Most physicians go into medicine to fulfill a calling with a burning desire to heal. We sacrifice greatly in the service of "our calling"—sacrificing our sleep, our youth, our relationships, our finances, and even ironically our health in this relentless pursuit to heal and deliver the best possible outcome for our patients. And I, like many of my kindred health care professionals, would argue that it would be worth it if it was really working. That is, after all, why we do it. But instead, we find ourselves thrust into an overwhelming environment and a situation that makes it impossible to make the healing difference that we envisioned as we went into medical school. Instead we find ourselves playing a game of hot potato with the patients in the hospital. And the evidence shows that it is not working—not at all. There is negative fallout from this beyond the patients. Medscape states that forty-two percent of all physicians report burnout and fifteen percent admit to depression. Physician suicide is over twice the national average of non-physicians and nearly triple in women physicians. There is a physician suicide every day in the U.S. with physicians having the highest suicide rate of any profession according to Medscape.

With extreme burnout rampant in health care workers and a rapidly increasing incidence of deadly—but potentially preventable—chronic disease, the increasingly important role of the health coach has emerged. As I became a certified health coach over a decade ago in addition to an M.D., I knew that if I could reach people and help them make those life changing lifestyle habits that I could make an even greater difference. A soul-satisfying difference. I had taken an oath as a medical doctor "to first do no harm." Knowing there were things I could do to help my patients avoid their needless suffering but being unable to effectively communicate this in the fast-paced medical system was "doing harm" in my opinion. It became unbearable—painful, even. It's impossible to alter a lifetime of unhealthy habits from a single doctor visit. This was the appeal of health coaching. I saw people transform through health coaching, but it took time! And it satisfied my soul.

I was not alone. Many others called to help this global health crisis sought ways to do this and grow a health coaching practice themselves. Unfortunately, most of these talented, well-meaning coaches failed to create a thriving practice. Especially as most coaches also had another job—often, though not always, burning them out in health care. They struggled with how to make a difference and a living with their own health coach program without putting their family and themselves at risk.

Is it really possible to have a rich, happy, soul satisfying life as a healer who truly makes a difference and still have time and money for yourself and your family?

Years ago, I thought this was an impossible dream. Many healers today are burned out, frustrated, overwhelmed, and stuck with a burning desire to heal but unable to actually fulfill this desire in a satisfying way. The original title for this book was "How Do I Get Out of My Soul-Sucking Life Alive?!" because that is exactly how I felt trapped in my suicide-inducing, lucrative medical career but still not fulfilling my calling to heal as I watched people destroy themselves every day. I endlessly struggled with the riddle: How do I leave my lucrative medical career to make a true healing difference in the world, without putting my family of six at risk, at a time when people weren't even looking to take responsibility for their own health? (They didn't even really appreciate they actually had a choice in their health.) I played the scenarios out many ways and the specifics of these choices always seemed to end disastrously for all.

Although it took me over a decade and over $100,000 to learn the lessons and come to the conclusions that I share in this book, it did not have to be that way. But I didn't know of another doctor or other health professional who had figured this out. I didn't even know if it was possible. There were no footsteps or roadmap to follow. I did have mentors (primarily single, male business mentors with no children and an occasional married business woman with an additional income stream from a partner), but no other medical or lucrative career they were considering leaving or a family they were putting at risk. There was certainly no one who would have been gutsy enough to dare to dream to leave a medical career at the top of their game to fulfill their soul's mission and find their happily ever after.

So, given my extreme situation, it was not surprising that my story would be inspirational to health coaches and other health professionals wondering how I did this "magic trick." I have many health coaches approaching me for "tips." But any answers that I could give in an email or a message would obviously be woefully inadequate. But as we look at the global health crisis and the critical role health coaches can play in reversing the tide, the answers are equally critical.

This book is in response to the many questions I received over the years, as doctors, nurses, health coaches, and other health professionals saw that I had actually broken away from my medical career to fulfill my soul's purpose to truly heal and make a difference. From their perspective, it seemed like some sort of magic trick or lucky break, but it wasn't that at all. Specifically, this book is in response to my client Nicole, who asked me how to create a signature health coaching program that would allow her to make a difference and a living. (Nicole now has an excellent program that helps women who have had bariatric surgery learn to eat healthy and love themselves so they can keep the weight off.) In retrospect, my journey (minus the errors of my years of trials) was actually a straightforward, repeatable specific Awakening Process™ that could be duplicated and that my clients now use to create their own successful signature programs.

This book will show you how to awaken to what you really want and how to do it without having to choose between making a living and living. You will know how to determine what influencers are sabotaging you and keeping you stuck. You will know how to easily implement simple baby steps that move you in the direction of your dreams. This book clearly outlines the nine step Awakening Process—the roadmap—that includes the necessary mechanics and mindset to create your own soul-satisfying signature program, allowing you to make a difference and a living doing what you love without putting your family at risk.

As Wayne Dyer said, "Don't die with your music inside." Imagine expressing your unique healing gift without sacrificing your life. But I know at the beginning of a journey how it feels to be trapped and uncertain and not see light at the end of your dark tunnel. Spoiler Alert: Everything is going to be okay. Breathe, and let me show you what I mean.

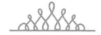

Chapter 1

My Awakened Healer Story

"Awakening is not changing who you are but discarding who you are not."

–Deepak Chopra

"I'm next! I am next!"

One crisp September morning in 2009 at St. Boniface Hospital in Canada, I was suddenly jolted awake. I'm next! I am next! I had been struggling to keep it together, feeling like I was always putting out fires, running from crisis to crisis, trying to keep up with everyone who needed a piece of me, knowing there just wasn't time for a full mental and physical breakdown which is what I craved. Even my computer got a refresh. Where the heck was mine? I was broken, fragile, vulnerable, just waiting for a cancer, heart attack, stroke, broken leg, or…something to take me out of the game and allow me to catch up. My mind occasionally flirted with horrible tragic extreme scenarios which would at least allow a reprieve…a coma? Imprisonment? Surely this would be better. "Stop the world and let me get off," I used to say. Or at least stop the world and let me catch up. I literally could not keep up with the desires I was launching for more ease, joy, love, support, relief.

I vividly remember that September morning working at the hospital as a subspecialty radiologist, standing in the sterile hallway, when I was told that not one but two colleagues—another radiologist and a family doctor that I had graduated medical school with—had committed suicide. Stunned, I went in to see my next patient who happened to be a doctor in whom I diagnosed a breast cancer! All of this that one September morning. I'm next! I'm next, I thought, if I don't change what I am doing! The signs were everywhere. I had seen the trajectory of unhealthy habits and killer stress in my patients and how that inevitably ended tragically, but here I was absolutely trapped in it myself. I knew I had to do something but the mountain I faced seemed insurmountable. I was sure there was no key to my golden handcuffs. I was trapped. We were chronically understaffed. At the time I was working full time as a doctor and every other week I was also on call twenty-four/seven. It was just not sustainable. I kept hanging in there because it kept "going to be better" but it just kept getting worse. But as docs, we were not going to get much sympathy making the great salaries that we did. Unfortunately working half as much for half the salary wasn't an option. The endless patients just kept coming. The workload obviously could not be cut in half and in fact, it kept increasing as I observed people daily destroy themselves in front of my eyes. Given that we were so understaffed, no radiologists in their right mind would be coming to join us and in fact, I wasn't the only one looking for a way out of the trap.

To the outside world, I had it made. A very "successful" medical career (the reason I had sacrificed and worked through seventeen years of post-secondary education of science and medical degrees, internship, and residencies), married with four healthy sons and a 6,000 square foot dream home along the river…what more could I possibly want? How ungrateful!

I had four beautiful sons that I had given birth to all within five- and three-quarter years of each other. Back in September 2009, they were six, eight, nine, and twelve years old. I loved them deeply but wondered why I had them if I could rarely see them…if I had to miss their Christmas mornings, their tuck-ins at night, their receiving awards, and many other milestones. When I dedicated my life to medicine and healing, I was prepared to make personal sacrifices, but I had not intended the enormous sacrifices that my decision was bestowing upon my future children. And what was this sacrifice for anyway? After decades into this game, I realized the hospital was one of the most difficult places to get any healing done. Was anyone actually being cured or were we just pin-balling people back and forth from test to test and specialist to specialist, slapping band aids on, measuring and categorizing lumps and bumps, before ultimately eventually admitting, "Sorry. There is nothing more we can do for you." (More on that later.)

My husband Gerald and I had been together since 1988 but now rarely saw each other awake. I was appreciative of the sacrifice that he had made to stay home and raise our four boys. This was a rare role reversal scenario we had embarked upon back in 1999, which came with its own challenges for him of navigating "mom and me" programs. There were definitely no other stay-at-home dads that we knew. But it just made sense to have at least one parent at home. But I still wanted to be "the mom." Their mom. As I would read the little duckling story to my boys, they would point to the mama duck and say, "Da Da!"...I couldn't help but have a twinge of pain, guilt, sadness rip through my body, but I was also grateful that they had a "Da Da" who was taking care of them and I swallowed that lump in my throat and moved on. I envied my stay at home mom friends. I did my absolute best to keep up with them. I volunteered for every school field trip and was present for every moment with my boys that I possibly could. I hosted the vast majority of large family dinners knowing how important family was but also knowing that my experience had taught me that if it is to be, it is up to me.

I became a master of squeezing forty-eight hours into twenty-four and being able to function on minutes rather than hours of sleep. I was exhausted from days to nights to days on call, driving home, and grabbing a quick micro nap at red lights. I couldn't see any other option. Definitely in need of sleep, I would have to get home first to make that dream of sleep come true. I remember one day fighting to stay awake on the drive home, fully caffeinated, windows down, radio blasting, focusing on the road ahead until I got home. Finally, as I pulled into our garage, I was able to relax... and hit the gas instead of the brake, lightly bumping into the tall shelving unit in our garage. It was a perfect metaphor for how I was living so close to the edge that it wouldn't take much for it all to come tumbling down.

I remember thinking back then, "Surely life can't get worse. Surely someone will save me. Surely someone will step in and say,

"You have suffered enough. We will take it from here. Thank you for what you have done. We won't add any more to your plate." But if you have ever given and given and given and given, assuming that sooner or later it will stop, then likely you too have realized there is no limit. It is a bottomless pit.

When I was thirty-seven weeks pregnant during my residency, I remember not wanting to ask my male colleagues for special favors and instead requesting in advance if I could do my share of call days earlier in my pregnancy rather than later. Of course, in my male-dominated specialty, no one could relate to why that might have been important and other priorities prevailed. So unfortunately, I actually had the most call of anyone in my third trimester while pregnant with my first son, being on call every second to third day with twenty-eight hour shifts and working full time in between. My legs were so swollen, I could barely fit shoes. I ended up having pre-eclampsia (pregnancy induced hypertension) with blurred vision and dizziness, forcing my first labor to be induced early. Not a great example of self-care nor care for my future family. But it is a great example of competing priorities and how there is no limit to what will be asked of you, if you allow it, which will inevitably result in the inability to take care of yourself or anyone else.

One of the biggest lessons I learned is that no one can really save you except for you. There is no knight in shining armor. No one else can sleep for you, eat for you, drink for you, move for you, think for you, believe for you…except you. But the great news is you can do it! You can heal yourself. So, this book is all about empowering you and showing you step by step how to "Be Good For You" and create your own soul-satisfying life. You will get to the point where you are so thankful for all of the trouble of this moment because it has forced you to see the only true solution that there ever was…and your life will forever be blissfully transformed! (I told ya that there is a happy ending after all, but we are just getting started here.)

How have I gotten myself into this mess? Have you ever wondered that? How did I get here? How did I fall into this trap … again!? And more importantly, how can I get myself out? That is what this book is all about. How can I get out of my soul-sucking life alive? And specifically as a healer, how can I break free to make a difference and a living doing soul-satisfying healing work? Whether you feel trapped in a horrible relationship, career, illness, financial situation, or any other stressful and massive dis-ease that feels impossible to get out of, I assure you, you can do this! I am living proof. The timeless core principles that I will be sharing with you are the same ones that I applied with my dad in 2016 when he had a massive stroke from which we were told he "could not survive." As a radiologist, as they showed me his scans, I knew what they were saying was medically correct. However, given my own personal journey and years of coaching and absolute knowing of our innate healing ability…what actually happened was he walked out of the hospital on his own two feet back home with my mom in a record thirty-five days! He was the Miracle Man. This amazing potential is within all of us. Wellness is who you really are! This is a message that deserves to be heard and will be laced throughout this book. But first, how did I fall into this trap?

When I was fourteen-years-old, my amazing grandmother died of cancer and I never wanted to see anyone have to experience that. So that event galvanized my lifelong mission to help people live their longest, healthiest, happiest lives. So, I went to medical school. Sounds logical. But twenty-five years as a doctor and I realized, that wasn't it. I was being paid extremely well to watch people destroy themselves in front of my eyes. Over seventy percent of everything I imaged as a radiologist, that kept us running into the hospital in the middle of the night, running in on call on Christmas morning, keeping us at the hospital instead of tucking in our babies, scanning someone instead of watching my son receive Athlete of the Year and everything that kept patients writhing in pain, fearing for their life—could have been prevented with a healthy lifestyle! I wanted to scream, "It doesn't have to be this way!" But given this crazy fast treadmill we were all on, I couldn't stop it while I was on it. The horrors I saw just kept coming.

I saw a forty-four-year-old woman that I diagnosed with not one but three cancers of the breast, ovary, and colon who was no longer a surgical candidate.

I saw a 400-pound man in I.C.U., wrapped in a bed sheet with terror in his eyes, so appreciative of the slightest kind gesture, but unseen as the nurses had to scurry around, attending to the machines ignoring the proverbial elephant in the room.

I saw a twenty-year-old obese, diabetic girl, sipping a Slurpee because she didn't feel right unless her sugars were sky high, who couldn't lay flat for her ultrasound, because her heart couldn't take it anymore.

Well, my heart couldn't take it anymore! I was no longer satisfied with being the "Official Photographer of Disease and Destruction!" But we were all trapped in this mess—not just me, but the other doctors, nurses, techs, admin staff, patients, all of us—running around, destroying our own health, destroying our own relationships … and it didn't have to be this way! That's why I made the big, bold move to go from the end of the line to the front lines to get out ahead of the impending doom and positively alter the fate of as many lives as I possibly could.

As a medical doctor for over twenty-five years, people kept giving their power away to me as their doctor so I could "fix" them. I think part of me wanted to "fix" people; that is why I became a doctor. But that is just not how it works. People have more power to impact their health than they realize through their choices. The body truly is the miracle that can heal itself if given half a chance. But, as Gandhi said, "Be the change you wish to see in the world." So, if I wanted a healthy, happy world, I had to clean up my own act first. I gave birth to my four sons in less than six years, and after each son, I would lose all but five pounds. That's not bad, but five pounds times four sons is twenty pounds, plus the ten I'd gained since high school. That's thirty pounds. I was overweight, sleep deprived, and we have also already established that I was immersed in our number one killer and the root of all dis-ease—Stress! My patients and colleagues were constant reminders of how that story ended, but I didn't know how to get out. Just stop. Stop what? My children? My income as the sole breadwinner? My patients? My family? My joy? My life?

Just what the heck was I supposed to stop? Although I didn't really want to die, I didn't know how to live. I was stuck. Trapped. And for any possible solution that you could have given me, I had more details of why that couldn't work and so there I was back and forth, back and forth, thoroughly stuck in my soul sucking life with no idea how to get out alive.

So, how did I? And more importantly, how can you? Well, like most turning points, my September morning didn't just happen out of the blue. There were a series of events, mini wake-up calls that led to the last straw and full awakening. Following my calling in those early days felt more like being prodded with a hot poker from behind rather than any spiritual quest. I would later learn this was because of my resistance to let go. I was already inadvertently building a parallel—or rather a separate, divergent life—in my quest for answers until ultimately, I had to make a choice of which path to follow and I definitely "took the one less travelled and that has made all the difference."

Wake-Up Call: Held Hostage in the Hot Tub

On spring break in 2004, we drove from our Manitoba home for the weekend to the Holiday Inn in Fargo, North Dakota. Our boys were just one, two, four, and six years old. (By the way, and not that it is anyone's business, but other than my first son whose conception was timed to when I would be exposed to the least amount of radiation, the latter three sons were conceived despite full contraception. What?! So, if you are thinking, "Well, she brought this all on herself," I would say, "Not intentionally…but absolutely, yes!" We all bring everything on ourselves. We create all of it. More on this later, too.)

Anyway, my husband and I had spent the day at the indoor hotel pool with the boys. We had a full day there and I wanted to sit in the hot tub for a bit before we went back to our room. Finally, a moment to relax. My wonderful husband occupied our boys by the pool. Of course, the boys were very little and getting restless. So, I was just about to get out of the pool when…dun…dun…duuunnn… in walks a male radiologist, from the same Canadian hospital I had trained as a resident at, with his family. Now remember, I still had my accumulated baby fat on me. In my younger years, I had worked hard to be fit and keep a lid on my weight…being Freshie Queen in high school, first runner-up for the Miss Blue Bomber Pageant, and second runner-up and Miss Congeniality in the Miss Winnipeg Pageant. So, in my teens and twenties, I wanted to look good. In my thirties when I started a family, I was at least thirty pounds overweight, sitting up to my shoulders literally in hot water in the hot tub. So as my colleague, who also knew me before kids, walked in—I gasped. The mental war began in my head.

"How could you let yourself go, Shaunna?"

"What do you expect? You've had four kids! It doesn't matter what you look like."

"Ugh! I know what I look like! I can't get out of the hot tub!"

"I have to get out of the hot tub."

I heard my boys say, "Come on, mom. Let's go! We're tired. Come on, mom!"

Ugh! By this time, I had been spotted by the other doctor. We smiled and nodded, acknowledging we saw each other from across the pool. He was on the opposite side with his family, and I was extremely grateful for the water up to my armpits covering my body, but I was starting to become a prune and my boys were becoming relentless. Ugh! I mean what are the chances?! Ultimately, I had to bite the bullet and get out of the pool and waddle my wet, overstuffed body over to the towels and cover up as quickly as I could.

That weekend I vowed never to be held hostage by my own body again. However, not for the reason you may think. Not because of how it looked to others or this other doctor, who almost certainly hasn't given that event as much thought as I have. But because of the simultaneous journey I was seeing my patients travel. If I didn't change, I would be going down the same path that landed them in the hospital. I had to first be the change I wanted to see. I knew that there were things I could do that were healthier. I knew knowing those choices and making those choices was easier said than done. But I also observed that I wasn't able to keep up with my four boys who were starting to play soccer, and I was getting winded just trying to keep up with them. I thought, this is no good. I need to be a better role model for my boys. I need to stay alive for my boys. I knew I was stressed. I knew I felt like I had no time. But my health is important, and I couldn't help my patients or my family if I couldn't help myself.

What Does It Mean to Be Truly Healthy?

I still remember driving back from that spring break weekend, eating a bag of Doritos (sometimes overhauling habits is gradual), inspired by my patients' poor examples and determined by personally being embarrassed and literally in hot water, I silently vowed to myself to be the absolute healthiest I could possibly be and live my longest, healthiest, happiest life—for me, for my children, and for all of the people who would follow in my footsteps. So that had me thinking: what does it mean to be truly healthy—physically, emotionally, financially, spiritually—in every way?

That moment. That decision and forward focus set into motion an incredible (eternal) quest to answer that question! I had a voracious appetite and read endlessly, devouring book after book and articles—I never left home without a book or an article to read. I discovered the power of influencers like superfoods and low glycemic magic foods and a whole wonderful world of wellness just waiting to be explored and enjoyed. It was like my decision and positive focus had unlocked a door to a new world of infinite wellness. With this shift in awareness, instead of trying to just fit into a skinny pair of jeans or fight my fat, this positive focus on health and positive changes that I could do, resulted in a thirty-pound healthy weight loss by

June! In less than three months, I had gone from hefty to hot, and I felt fantastic! More importantly, I realized that it wasn't hard. It was actually surprisingly easy and fun despite years of struggling with my weight in my teens. I thought everyone should know this. But I knew no one would believe how important the mindset and identity shift were. In fact, many people wrongly assumed I had starved myself or worked out at the gym. In fact, the ease of it was the missing ingredient for me in the past and is the missing ingredient for most people. The struggle and the fight were and are actually part of the problem. It was astounding to me! This doesn't have to be hard! Ease is the key!

As I gradually became more aware and awakened to this core truth, watching my patients suffer needlessly became even more unbearable because now I really knew that it didn't have to be this way. But also, I realized that the power lay within themselves and their choices. In the hospital, ironically it just wasn't the time or place to show or tell people how to be healthy. Patients were not for the most part ready to hear the great news that they had the power to massively impact their health through their choices because that would also mean, the bad news—that their choices had led them to their current situation. I should add that this is not about blame or fault. Obviously, no one wants to be sick. No one really wants to feel bad. But our health and state of well-being is our responsibility and when we know better, we can do better. As Maya Angelou says, "Do the best you can until you know better. Then when you know better, do better."

The next ten to fifteen years was a time of great discovery, awakening, and refining of my process. The first thing I wanted to do was share the immense power of lifestyle choices with the world. But I was still also immensely stressed and trapped in the golden handcuffs of my medical career. I remember sitting on the open staircase in my dream home along the river, looking out at the view, tears rolling down my face as I gazed upon my beautiful custom kitchen, gorgeous hardwood floors, and treasured one-of-a-kind light fixtures, and my beautiful front door and thinking: I absolutely love this home—my baby. I truly do. Not for anyone else. I don't care what others think of this. But I love this. I helped design and pick out every window and door knob. This home was years in the making and I absolutely love it…but not more than I love myself. If I wanted to take a stand for my patients and help them truly be proactive and dedicate my time and energy to truly helping people be healthy, I could not keep this. I could not afford to keep this going without running endlessly on the treadmill which led to nowhere.

But how could I leave my lucrative medical career and still make a difference healing without putting my family at risk? I did not know anyone who had ever done this. That night a late-night desperate web search led me to Deepak Chopra and also the Institute for Integrative Nutrition (IIN). Their words, missions, and philosophies aligned perfectly. I remember thinking—Yes! Yes! This is what I am talking about. There was (as Canadian musician Leonard Cohen alludes to) a slight crack in my perfect facade where the light could get in. I saw a ray of hope. I eagerly enrolled in their programs simultaneously to learn as much as I possibly could about how to get my message to the world.

One of the first transformational events was Deepak's *Journey into Healing*. I went to learn how to heal others but of course, what happened was I began to awaken, shift my perspective, and heal myself. At another Chopra event, Deepak was talking about archetypes and how we all have within us the hero, the victim, the saboteur, the prostitute, etc. I remember raising my hand and telling him, "I'm a prostitute." Immediately heads turned around from people sitting in front of me with shocked looks upon their face. I repeated. "I'm a prostitute. I mean my profession is a medical doctor, but I am absolutely miserable. I wanted to heal people but that isn't really what is happening and if I am honest about it—if I am so miserable why don't I quit? It's for the money. I never went into medicine for the money. There are many easier ways than this to make money. But if I don't really like it and I am forcing myself to pretend I like it and I am still doing it for the money—I'm a prostitute."

Deepak and I discussed this for a few minutes, and we talked about different archetypes that I (people) could choose to identify from mythology like Athena or other mythical or even real people, past or present. To which I asked Deepak, "Can I be Wonder Woman?" "Yes. You can be Wonder Woman," Deepak replied. It sounds silly but adorning an empowering identity albeit fictitious instead of a disempowering identity was significant. As I write this, I am looking at the Wonder Woman lunch box in my office on my shelf as a little reminder of the power, strength and focused powerful femininity embodied in this heroine. If you look at many pictures of me on my drshaunna.com website or old photos or videos, it is not uncommon to see bracelets on both of my wrists—my secret little nod and acknowledgment of the Wonder Woman in me that was going to be required to show up if I was going to be the heroine of my own story.

I enrolled in Integrative Nutrition (the world's largest nutrition school) and became a certified holistic health coach. When I went there, the program consisted of live classes in New York. I would fly straight from the hospital on a Friday night after work, get to my hotel in the wee hours and make my way to the event first thing Saturday morning. I'd attend classes all day Saturday and Sunday and fly back Sunday night to Winnipeg, Canada so I could be at the hospital by 7:00 a.m. to scan the breast patients before the regular scans started at 8:00 a.m. I was on call every second or third week and these New York trips were also every second or third week.

So, for months I was either at the hospital, on call or in New York. My boys were still little, and I couldn't have done this if my husband hadn't chosen to stay home with our boys. This was a hard time but also a magical time in New York. I was learning and awakening to a new way of looking at health. It embodied what I had come to know and believe but it was wonderful to know I was not alone. It was wonderful to be there with 1,000 to 2,000 other health coaches in training learning how we could really make a difference coaching people to healthy habits. Joshua Rosenthal is the amazing visionary who founded this school twenty years ago and I will be forever grateful for his creation of this program and movement that allowed me to have the structure to bring what I knew in my heart could help so many people. As I went through the curriculum and experienced the community, I became even more aware of the magnitude of our global health crisis. Where does one even begin?

Wake-Up Call: Wake Up!

One Saturday morning I was sleeping, exhausted from a previous week on call when my youngest son Brennan came into my room.

"Come on, mom. Come on, mom. Wake up. Let's play."

"Um. Uh. Okay, Brennan. Okay. Just give me a few more minutes and then I'll wake up."

Then out of the mouths of babes, he said, "What if you don't even know how to wake up?"

That got me up! That woke me up! What if I don't even know how to "wake" up? What if society doesn't even know how to wake up?! That is the problem. We don't even know how to wake up and stop this crazy train wreck. I had been ignoring several wake-up calls all along the way that were attempting to gently nudge me onto my soul fulfilling path. My van on my way to work had the anti-lock brake light on saying "trac off." It would be a year later when it would dawn on me that I was off track! The smokers at the hospital were supposed to smoke outside far from the hospital building but in the frigid Manitoba winters, the staff (ironically from oncology), would just go outside the back door—right near an intake vent. An intake vent that led the cigarette smoke right through to the vent over my chair in my office where I sat and read films all day in ultrasound. The universe was even trying to smoke me out of my literally toxic environment! In retrospect, I was missing all of these wake-up calls! We all are. So how could we wake up? *What could we do? What could I do?* That is the answer. Looking at what you can do. Focusing positively in the direction you want and taking those baby steps. This is a very important piece in The *Awakening* Process and a very important factor in my dad's miraculous recovery from his "fatal" stroke that would happen almost a decade later. Start small in the right direction and scale from there.

I began to see clients in my home one by one. This was tremendously satisfying. At one point all of my clients were off all of their medications. I did not take them off. Their doctors took them off. But as these clients cleaned up their diet, lost weight, had support, and knew how to make some gradual and yet ultimately powerful lifestyle shifts, amazing things happened. They were getting energized. They had renewed purpose and joy. I was waking up too.

Wake-Up Call: What Do I want?

Another powerful exercise again at a Chopra event occurred when I was meditating, and we were supposed to ask ourselves, "What do I want? What do I really want?" I had no clue. No idea. I knew clearly what I did not want—my current life. But I had no idea as to what I *did* want. So, I closed my eyes and casually, still feeling lost like this was a bit of a waste of time, I thought, "What do I want? Hmmm. Let's see. Umm. What—do—I—want?"

And then it happened. Out of nowhere, someone's pager went off. No one was supposed to have cell phones or pagers in the room; but there it was. The exact same beep as my hospital pager that had haunted me for decades now. The shrill and triggering *Beep! Beep! Beep!* Tears streamed uncontrollably down my face. My face got red. My heart started to race, and I breathed heavily, and it was suddenly crystal clear. I don't ever want to be on effing call again! Not ever. Never! Ever! I feel like the universe or God, or however you want to look at this, was laughing a little and saying, "There. Now that wasn't so difficult was it?"

So, for the first time I actually started to consider a life without call, something I didn't even dare to dream before. I started now to consider: Well, what do I want? I wanted to work three days a week, no evenings, no call, make a wonderful healing difference, be appreciated for what I did…and while we are at it since all that was impossible—make bucketfuls of money. I mean why not? That was an impossible dream so might as well add that in. It was illegal for us to do ultrasound outside of the hospital in Manitoba where I worked so that meant full-time call even if I chose to go part time. So, it didn't matter. Might as well say what I wanted. And within a year that impossible dream had come true! One of many "impossibles" to become possible that was yet to come. Positive focus in the direction you want, regardless of reality or odds, is very, very powerful!

With a new part-time position in a Calgary ultrasound clinic, I had more flexibility with my time, and I could grow my coaching practice when I was not in Calgary. The flights to work were challenging, but I wrote a large part of my first book *Doctor up the Recipe* on that plane. Ironically, I saw my kids more, even though I worked two provinces away, than I did when I worked in my local hospital. With no TV or friends and minimal furniture in my Calgary condo that I stayed in, I read and listened to podcasts and educational audios and fueled my mind continuously. Various aspects of my health coaching practice gradually increased—speaking, writing, workshops, coaching and even taking on a product partner that aligned with my philosophies and later a medical device—both of which would later prove instrumental in my dad's recovery. As this increased, I gradually phased out my clinic hours, initially flying in to mainly do procedures and then ultimately just two days a week every other week and then as the flights, car rentals, and hotel bookings and security pat downs grew wearisome just to go to work, I eventually left my clinical practice.

The transition was not like a checkered flag finish line or a flag that I planted at the top of my mountain when I reached the summit. It wasn't like that at all. Instead with intense focus on the direction that I was going, I kept my head down and kept working and working and inching and inching in the positive direction of my destination of what I wanted, continually refining what that was. Choosing to focus on what was working. Ignoring to the best of my ability the many things that weren't. Continually focused with my head down in the positive direction until one day I looked up and realized—I was here. I was now at my happily ever after. I was living in my dream location in beautiful Kelowna, BC, Canada in a beautiful home with a beautiful family that I got to see every day. I was living with my amazing husband of twenty-five years that I got to walk the dog with whenever we wanted. I got to coach clients that I adore and inch them toward their happily ever after.

Beyond that, there have been other perks; I get to speak on large stages in front of thousands and inspire the masses on healthy living. I inspire health coaches to be the best version of themselves and to keep going and make the difference they were born to make—to be the change they wish to see. To answer their wake-up call. I had fully awakened my inner healer and I was finally free to heal.

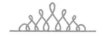

Chapter 2

Solving the Impossible

"After every storm the sun will smile; for every problem there is a solution, and the soul's indefeasible duty is to be of good cheer."
–William R. Alger

W hat I eventually realized was the years of struggle was not a necessary part of the solution. What was actually required was a paradigm shift. Then it was like flipping a switch that brought greater clarity with the light, allowing things to move swiftly into place. That is my goal for you. I want to turn on your light switch so you can shine your light brightly and the world will be a much brighter, healthier, happier place. I can't do this alone. The world needs you. In this book, we will dive deep into the core of this paradigm shift that allows you to solve the unsolvable, make possible the impossible and that which is the basis of miracles. Eldridge Cleaver may have inspired the famous quote, "If you are not part of the solution, you are part of the problem," but I have come to discover that *if you are not part of the problem, you are part of the solution.*

Now as I gradually became more aware and *awakened* to this core truth and directed my attention away from the problem and toward the positive solution, incredible transformations happened. Having coached thousands of people now to successful transformation including myself and my dad's miraculous stroke recovery, this process has become simultaneously more simplified and more powerfully transformative over time. However, as I look back at how far this process has evolved, I know that if I jump in with you at the punch line, you will miss the power of this completely and may dismiss this as wishful or positive thinking. Consider this analogy. People thousands of years ago believed the world was flat because as they looked around, they saw plenty of evidence to confirm their view of the flat earth. If someone was to just jump to the punch line and share their new truth that the world was round, they were going to—at the very least—be called insane and dismissed, if not worse.

In fact, it took thousands of years for people to come to accept this idea of a round earth put forth by visionaries who shared evidence to back up this new perspective after seeing flaws with the flat earth viewpoint despite appearances. So, throughout this book, as I make the case for the fact that you absolutely can heal your life, *you*—yes, *you*—really can create your own signature program that can make a difference and allow you to make a living to support your family without putting your family at risk.

Some of you who are facing some impossible looking situations may be tempted to believe in what you see. You may believe "the world looks flat; the tests showed I have…; it's impossible to leave my career." This would be a tragic mistake of epic proportions to not even consider the bigger picture and the more profound truth that who you really are is pure wellness. This is the basis of the secrets of self-healing that I also love to teach which you will glean throughout this book as a bonus. I believe in informed consent. I believe in education. I believe in giving people information and allowing people to make up their own opinions. My goal is not to convince you of anything. But rather, my goal is to show you what I have learned over more than fifty years and especially over the past twenty-five years and especially over the past five years. So that if you too feel like all hope is gone or you live in fear that something awful is about to happen, that you can learn through what follows about what is possible, become inspired, believe it can happen for you and take the simple steps to create your program as you go through this book.

The *Awakening Process*™ is a nine-step program that simultaneously builds you the confident healer and holistic entrepreneur as you build your program. It is customized to you to awaken your inner healer. We want your program to be an extension of who you really are. That will be authentic. That will satisfy your soul. That will attract the ideal clients that you are meant to serve. That will transform. "Done for you" programs are great perhaps if you are just starting out but there is a reason that you want to heal and help others. Often in my experience, health coaches and healers have a story—something that they have overcome, that causes them to be a powerful crusader for the people they are meant to serve. If I hadn't gone through my story, I would not be so passionate and committed to my clients to deliver their very best results. It feels amazing to truly make this difference. Your results will begin to speak for themselves and you will be in ease and flow and can be in a position like myself, where you can pick and choose who you want to work with from the people that are *coming to you*. This is very different than hunting clients. This program is love-based. It comes from love not fear. It will deliver the concrete mechanics to get it done as well as the critical mindset to allow this to flow to you and sustain it. You will want to have a notebook handy as you go through the steps. Do the exercises in this book as you go because each step builds toward your signature program. In this book, you will learn the *Awakening Process* and will know how to:

Awaken to your soul's purpose: How to get crystal clear on what you really want.

Who can you serve: How to get crystal clear on your ideal client and your niche.

Align your program to be the best solution: Learn the secret to leverage your time and become world class and deliver the best results for your client.

Keep inching forward with baby steps: With clarity on who you serve and how you serve, you will start to test your messaging and program idea from a place of love.

Elevate yourself to your soul's purpose: You will learn a powerful tool to elevate you to your confident, clear, loving, best version of yourself and the strategies to overcome sabotage.

Name the steps in your signature program: Your program begins to take shape as you outline the steps to take your client from their specific problem to their specific solution.

Identify Your Influencers: You will understand the immense power of influencers and how to consciously choose your best influencers to lead to your success and avoid self-sabotage.

Nurture your clients and yourself. You will learn how a soul satisfying signature program nurtures you and your client and the clean role money plays in this relationship.

Grow yourself; grow your movement. You will learn the attractive archetypes and the identity shift required to lead a successful signature program and your movement.

By the conclusion of this book, by using the Awakening Process, you will know how to create your own soul-satisfying wellness program that allows you to make a difference and a living and allows you to fully awaken your inner healer and be free to heal. Let's go solve the unsolvable, shall we?! Grab a pen and let's go!

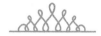

Chapter 3

Awaken to Your Soul's Purpose

"Every human being has a gift of genius and a personal calling encoded within them from birth. It is up to you to find it, to develop it and share this gift with the world. This is your life purpose."
–Oprah Winfrey

The first step in creating a soul-satisfying signature program is to get clear on what that means to you. What would satisfy your soul? What is your purpose? What are you meant to do? Because there are many ways to serve people and make a difference but not all of them are going to be truly satisfying. For example, I served many people with my medical career and it did make a difference, but it was not satisfying my deep core desire to truly heal and touch another person's soul. Each of us has a calling whether we can hear it or not. Just like the missed wake-up calls that I shared in Chapter

1, in retrospect you will see that there have been incidents and experiences that have been nudging you along and calling you to a more satisfying existence.

There is certainly more than one right answer and you can and will change your mind as you learn, grow, and evolve, and you literally are always on your path. Everything has and will shape you into the person you are and the person you will become, even experiences that you might be tempted to judge as negative (especially those ones). But as you embark on this journey, put your heart and soul into your signature program, and climb this mountain together, let's make sure we are climbing the right mountain! I spent seventeen years of postgraduate training and twenty-five years as a medical doctor (some overlap of years) to get to the top of my game and climb to the tippy top of that mountain only to realize…uh oh…wrong mountain. It was a lot harder with all of the time, money and energy that was invested into that to start to climb another mountain in my forties and arguably as the sole breadwinner, potentially to place my family at risk. But as the sole income earner, I was really looking to be a soul income earner. So, if you want to create the life of your dreams—let's create the life of your dreams!

When I was faced with this pivotal moment and trying to decide what did I really want to do with my life, I found inspiration from Deepak Chopra's instruction as he taught me to meditate. He had our group ask ourselves these three questions as we went into meditation:

1. Who am I?
2. What do I want?
3. How can I serve?

Now, the point really wasn't to come up with labels as to who we were or even to answer the questions at all but rather just to ask and then meditate and quiet the mind. Let me just speak about meditation for a moment.

I am not sure whether you have ever meditated, have a regular meditation practice, or if you think it is a great idea but can't seem to fit it into your busy schedule or if you think it is far too "woo-woo" or out there for you, but this is actually really important. If you have a regular meditation practice that is working for you, then keep up the great work. Otherwise, just know that I fit all of the previous descriptions before I established my meditation practice. Meditation is so subtle it seems like you are doing "nothing," but it makes all the difference in the world! I was told that it takes twenty-one days to make a habit. I am not sure if that is actually true, but I can tell you it took me five years to meditate twenty-one days in a row! So, I get it if you are busy and life is crazy but all the more reason to fit it in. Here are some tips that have worked for me and any meditation or stillness practice is better than none.

The point of meditation is to quiet your mind and tune into your inner being, your higher self, your soul, infinite intelligence, source, God, or whatever label you like for this. Unlike prayer where you are asking, in meditation you are listening.

So, find a comfortable place and time to quiet your mind. For me, first thing in the morning, I set my alarm sixteen minutes early and I meditate most often in bed. It does help to sit up, so you don't fall asleep, but if you fall asleep (especially in the early days), it is probably a sign that you need the sleep. I also have a nice armchair in my room by a window that is another favorite spot.

Deepak recommends twenty minutes twice a day, and that is just not something that I could seem to do back in those early days. As you will learn throughout this book, what I did do was *focus on what I could do*. So, what I could do was fifteen minutes first thing in the morning. I would set my alarm—like a snooze alarm—only I would sit up and meditate instead of rolling over back to sleep. I gave myself an extra minute to get set up.

Next, I closed my eyes and asked myself those three questions. A mantra is often recommended, and you can certainly do that. "So-Hum" is a popular one that corresponds with your in and out breath. But also, what I found worked well was to listen to "nothing"—what I mean by that is that I would focus on the hum of the furnace or air conditioner in the background or I would turn on the bathroom fan and focus on that. Sometimes I google white noise and meditate to YouTube audios of white noise. Another practical tip is that I actually stare at the back of my eyelids. I know this sounds funny. But if I didn't focus on looking at the blank dark canvas that is the back of my eyelids and if I just closed my eyes, my mind would wander to my never-ending to-do lists, and my meditations wouldn't really be quieting my mind. So, these are some little tips to get you started if you haven't yet. Meditation will change your life and is probably the best way I can serve you by getting you hooked up to you.

Meditation is an excellent way to awaken to your soul's purpose, but often when I am working with health professional clients, they appreciate something more active that they can do to get them pointed in the right direction. If you haven't done so yet, grab a pen and a journal and ask yourself these eight questions (that purposefully overlap each other):

1. When have I felt the most alive and happy?
2. When have I felt the best about myself?
3. What do I love to do?
4. What do others say I am good at?
5. What are my natural gifts, strengths and characteristics?
6. How do I like to interact with people (online versus live, group versus one-on-one, etc.)?
7. What am I most passionate about?
8. How would I change the world if I could?

Next, look at your answers and see if you can pick out a theme and intersections that are apparent between what you love to do, what you are excellent at and that fit with how you want to change the world. Don't stress if nothing is obvious at the moment. Just asking the question is helpful and brings awareness to what you want and then you may have an "aha" moment like I did when the pager went off during a meditation on the question "What do I really, really want?" bringing crystal clarity to an answer that I (and you may have) felt forbidden to allow. After all what right did I as a medical doctor, who had dedicated her life to helping people heal, have to want to see my children, be with my husband and not work evenings, weekends or on call and still find a way to make a difference healing?

Another question that I ask all of my clients whether they are health professionals looking to create their signature program or a busy mom looking to lose weight, is the "Magic Wand" question. So, if I have a magic wand and you go to sleep tonight and I wave this magic wand and you wake up living your ideal dream life, what does it look like? In this fantasy world you can be, do, have anything and it does not have to be based in reality. You can wear fairy wings on the moon if that is what you want. In this exercise, there are no limits on your time, finances, emotions, relationships or geography. You can have anything. Where are you living? Who are you with and what are you doing? Take a moment to write this down now. Do it. Because each step builds upon the previous and we want to make sure we are climbing your right mountain. Make sense? Cool.

Most people have long since buried their dreams or put them on a high up dusty shelf. Now is the time to dust that off and make your dreams come true. We are not going to be creating just any ol' program here. We are going to be creating *your* soul-satisfying signature program! So, the next thing we want to consider is what is the specific outcome that you want from your program? Is this a part-time or full-time venture for you? Are you trying to find a way to leave a lucrative medical career but still make a difference healing? If so, how much would you like to earn in the next year, that would allow your signature program to be your "soul" income? Just like we are going to get super specific on how and who you serve, we want to get super specific on what you want and cast the vision for that. The vague idea to "help everyone be healthier" is doomed right from the start.

But when you create a destination you are trying to reach it becomes almost magical how life can conspire on your behalf when you are doing your soul's work. It will often feel like there is a larger force than you at work and you are just playing your part. This is exactly how I felt when I helped my dad recover from his "fatal" stroke. There were so many "strokes of luck" (the subject of another book) that I just played my part and there was a clarity and ease about it. I had the same feeling when I created the first beta group to help health coaches create their signature programs after *they came to me.* This is the way we want your program to feel for you. Your signature program is such an extension of who you really are and how you are meant to serve that you are excited, enthused and passionate about it and you wake up every day on fire about the people you get to serve! There is no monetary value that equates to this feeling.

However, we also have mortgages to pay and mouths to feed and if we don't find a way to fund our movement, then we stay stuck at our day job and don't make the difference or live the life we were meant to live. We will talk more about pricing and when and if you actually want to quit your day job in Chapter 10; for now, how much would you like to earn in the next year that would be good for you? Pick a number. It can be changed but we want to have a destination to put on your map. Then divide that number by twelve to get your desired monthly income for this to make sense for you. Then put that aside for now. As we go through the process, I will demonstrate how to get there.

As we revisit the three questions at the beginning of the chapter, "Who you are" is not even something that has an answer that can be spoken. But I want you to own the essence of who you really are which is pure wellness and quite frankly awesome! That is who you really are! The third question "How can I serve?" is with your soul-satisfying signature program. So that leaves us with "What do I want? What do I really, really want?" The exercises in this chapter will assist you to gain clarity around this.

To light your path even further, I am super excited to share with you the *BGOOD4U Awakening Map*™ which is an excellent tool that I share with my clients to help them get from point A to point B. I want you to imagine (or better yet, draw in your journal) a horizontal line in the middle of your page. Then in the middle of the page draw a vertical line so you have a large "+" on your page. On the right-hand side of the horizontal line, write Positive Direction. On the left-hand side of the horizontal line, write Negative Direction. Now in the right upper quadrant write *Love* and in left lower quadrant write *Fear*. In the bottom left corner of your page write "Dis-ease" and the top right corner of your page write "Ease." But also, in this top right corner put "B" (as in we are going to move from point A to B) and also put *Pure Wellness* which is who you really are. These are the basics of your map that you are going to continually reference as we walk through the *Awakening Process*.

Let's fill it in. Starting at the left-hand side of your page just below the horizontal line, I want you to write a list of emotions (states of consciousness) starting with Courage, Pessimism, Frustration, Overwhelm, Disappointment, Doubt, Worry, Blame, Anger, Revenge, Jealousy, Unworthiness, Fear, Grief, Apathy, Depression, Guilt and ending with Shame in the bottom left corner.

Before moving to the upper half, write along the horizontal line: Boredom to the left of midline and Neutral to the right of midline. Along the far-right margin, write the following moving upward above the horizontal line: Satisfaction, Willingness, Optimism, Belief, Enthusiasm, Passion, Love, Joy, Freedom, and Enlightenment in the far upper right corner.

I would like to acknowledge the work of Dr. David Hawkins in his calibration of the levels of consciousness in *Power vs. Force*, and also the work of Esther, Jerry, and Abraham Hicks for their work on the Emotional Guidance Scale as outlined in *The Amazing Power of Deliberate Intent* that were inspirational for me in creating the *BGOOD4U Awakening Map*.

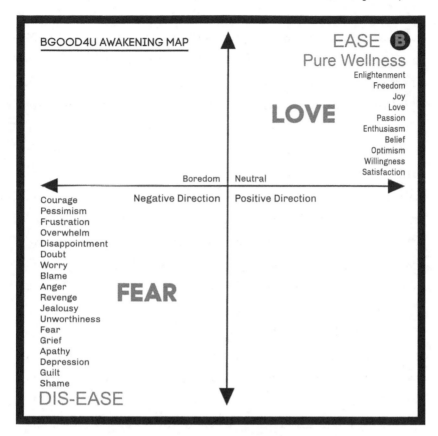

So, now that you have this map, how do we use it? This map is a great visual of something I have learned over the years and can be summed up with the phrase I've heard Abraham say, "You can't get there from there." So, we want to put your destination—what you have determined what you really, really want—up at the top right corner. Put it right up there at love, joy, freedom, and enlightenment because happiness is why we do everything and what we really, really want.

What I discovered over decades of working harder and harder, and struggling more and more, and getting more and more frustrated and overwhelmed or even angry or jealous or guilty is that I could not get to my promised land from there. Even though I was told by others to work harder or suffer more and even though I became the queen of delayed gratification—there was no joy at the end of that miserable road. No one was ever going to say, "Oh, my goodness! Look how much you have suffered?! Here you go—everything you want is now yours. All your dreams have come true." Nope. That never happened. That never happens. As I have said before, the only person who can really save you is—*you*. However, when I focused *forward in the positive direction of what I did want*, and took the *baby steps* in the *positive direction*, my results happened faster than I could ever have possibly imagined!

Now this may seem hokey to you, and that is okay, but I promise you it is not! This right here can have life-changing and lifesaving implications and is the exact same process (in addition to the other tools I will share in this book) that I used to help my dad recover from his stroke.

So, in the summer of 2016, my eighty-two-year-old dad suffered a massive stroke which the doctors told us he could not survive. They said he would not recognize us, and it was far too massive and there was nothing that they could do for him and they transferred him to the community hospital to die. The doctors showed me his scans, and as a medical doctor of twenty-five years and especially as a radiologist, I knew what they were saying was medically correct from their perspective. But I also knew from working as a health coach for over a decade that who we really are is pure wellness (Point B on the map), and that we can tap into that with focus in the *positive direction*, taking *baby steps* in the direction of *what we want*. So, my focus was counter intuitive for most. I came from love not fear. I focused on what I could do, not on what I couldn't do. I focused on what I did want, not on what I didn't want. I took a one-way ticket home to see my dad not knowing if I would make it in time for him to be alive. I purposely did not pack a black dress. I definitely did pack and read a book by Dr. Norman Doidge entitled *The Brain's Way of Healing* on the plane because I could not sleep anyways. I became so inspired from that book that by the time I landed, I just needed my dad to have a pulse. I knew I could work with anything else. I knew the brain was a use-it-or-lose-it organ— that early on could be rewired and recruited to take over tasks. So, focusing on any slightest sensation or movement that he did have was key. In other words, positively focusing on what he could do rather than what he couldn't do. If we had a little, we could have more. This is the same approach I recommend to coaches building their business. Start small. Find something that works. Then scale upward from there.

During my dad's hospital stay when I was told a horrible prognosis or bad news, I did not fight back nor tell them they didn't know what they were talking about nor defiantly say "I'll show you!" I did not go to the angry, frustrated, overwhelmed, or blaming side of the map. Instead, I just let their words pass right through me without sticking, lovingly knowing that everyone is always doing the best they possibly can from where they are. As we go through the *Awakening Process*, I will reference my dad's story where relevant. But it's important that you know now that through this work, coming from love, my dad walked out of there on his own two feet. He was back home with my mom in a record thirty-five days, defying all the odds—earning him the title Miracle Man! The day my dad went home from the hospital, there was a woman half his age with half as severe a stroke who was just starting to stand. This is the power of what I am sharing here—of positive focus, taking baby steps in the direction of what you want!

It is really important that we know what you want so we can focus on it rather than perhaps your current situation. What is your point B? Do the exercises in this chapter and get clear on this. As you keep asking over the next few weeks it will become clearer. But make a point of focusing on what you do want rather than on what you don't want and upon what is working not on what isn't working. I appreciate this is easier said than done but it makes all the difference in the world!

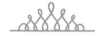

Chapter 4

Who Can You Serve?

"The best way to find yourself is to lose yourself in the service of others."

–Mahatma Gandhi

Now that we are gaining some clarity on what you want and awakening to your soul's purpose, we are starting to see how you can serve in a satisfying way in your signature program. So, the next question which is the most important question of the whole process is who can you serve? Once you know who you can serve, that will help to fill in the details as to how you can *best* serve your ideal client with your signature program. If you are a coach, then you already have heard the importance of a niche and the value of being an expert at solving a specific problem. You may have heard the phrase "the riches are in the niches" or something to that effect. We are going to take this idea to a whole other level to get your results to a whole other level!

Firstly, a medical career is vastly different than being a health coach or holistic entrepreneur. As a medical doctor, there is no shortage of patients. The emergency rooms, wards and waiting rooms are full of them. People know where to go if they are sick. They go to a hospital or a clinic. There is an entrance to the building. There is a phone number to book an appointment. Patients also know the routine. They know that they will show up—eventually get seen, state their specific problem, and the doctor will deliver some sort of specific result. The doctor may write a prescription, order some further tests, refer you to a specialist or reassure you, and send you on your way.

But as a health coach, you are at the forefront of a revolution in health care. People don't really know what you do or why they would see you or how it actually works. Health coaching is a very new line of work, and at the moment it is in the realm of entrepreneurship. I believe many health coaches with a desire to heal feel that they will just get their certification and then they will magically get hired like a dietician at the hospital or like a massage therapist in a wellness center. They don't realize they have just become an entrepreneur. This is why unfortunately many of these amazing people with a heart of service who are so knowledgeable and caring usually fail in their business and never do the soul-satisfying work they are meant to do. They don't really understand they are in business and if they do, most business advice isn't geared to people who want to be of service in a loving, soul-satisfying, healing way. This is why I am so passionate about this and writing this book. So many coaches want to make a difference and people are literally dying for their help, but the health coaches and clients can't find each other hiding in the jungle.

So, in order for potential clients to see you, hear you, and find you, your messaging has to be crystal clear and speak specifically directly to them...and, in fact, has to speak specifically directly to one person to solve one problem and deliver one result with your one business. That is the secret sauce right there! Hardly anyone does this. I learned this the trial and error and error and error way and fortunately in the early days, I had a medical career to bank roll this costly mistake that takes most health coaches out of the game right at the starting gate. It is a trap for healers. We want to heal everyone from their everything and in doing that we heal no one and stay stuck at our day job and get sick in the process. It is a tragic tale told thousands of times a day every day.

It doesn't have to be this way. A better destination on your map to focus on is to become the absolute best in the world in your specific niche! Well if you are just starting out and feeling confused and uncertain, how the heck do you do that?! Well, through *positive focus, taking baby steps, in the direction that you want* but let me show you.

As a medical doctor, I specialized in radiology (diagnostic imaging) and eventually specialized in ultrasound. Then following areas of interest and also in response to need and unanswered questions, I specialized further in interventional ultrasound and especially in breast, thyroid, and eventually foot ultrasound. I know that seems random, but as a new radiologist, I specialized in ultrasound because I actually liked the patient contact and blending the art and science of scanning and problem solving. When I started, hardly anyone was doing breast ultrasound, and the department head took me under her wing and mentored me in those early days—mainly because she was overrun with patients and needed the help. Being a woman in a male-dominated specialty and helping women in the sensitive area of breast ultrasound also helped. Soon we had so many patients that would come even from out of province to see us. We would scan women before work at 7 a.m., through our lunch hour, and after work. We were a referral center without any sign that said so. We ended up creating teaching cases to teach other radiologists and technologists in North America how to scan and interpret these scans. It was a very specific area and we did it a lot. We got great at it and word got out and we definitely didn't need to advertise.

As assistant professor of medicine in diagnostic imaging, I was teaching other radiologists and technologists during our monthly province-wide rounds. I needed to come up with a topic one month. I didn't know a lot about thyroid ultrasound, and, quite frankly, I didn't know many people who did. We knew the basics, but the basics still left me with unanswered questions and not feeling confident and satisfied that we were giving patients and referring doctors actual useful information and guidance. So, I decided to teach this. This forced me to learn it well from whatever research was out there among world leaders. After all, someone in the world must know these answers and have done the studies.

As I distilled this research into practical useful algorithms and an approach for myself and other radiologists and technologists, suddenly I was now the expert. Now I was being referred people from elsewhere in the city and province. I was getting the really hard cases, which forced me to get even better, knowing there wasn't anywhere else for me to refer these people. There is another teaching gem in this example and that is speak on a specific subject. Know all that you can. Share that information. Become the world expert. By speaking, others can tell you are expert at your niche, and they will follow you to the solution that only you can deliver in the way you deliver.

One final example is from the ultrasound clinic in Calgary where I was one of just three radiologists. The senior head doctor knew the value of niche focus and answering unanswered problems. His focus was vascular and musculoskeletal ultrasound and specifically, he began scanning patients with foot pain from Morton's neuroma. This is a very painful benign nodule between the toes that otherwise was left to the much more costly and less readily available MRI modality. He got highly skilled at detecting these with a special probe and taught me and the other radiologist how to detect these. We, then began successfully treating these with injections over a series of four appointments, much to the delight of our patients who could not find relief anywhere else. Soon we had patients coming from provinces away to our clinic to be seen and treated. I remember talking to a patient from Victoria, BC who had come to our Calgary clinic. I wondered how she had possibly found us. There was no bulletin. There were no Facebook ads. No website. There were no ads or testimonials celebrating our success at all! Word-of-mouth referrals about our specific tiny area of expertise once again attracted people from miles around.

So, the key is to be world class! I was not the best medical doctor or best radiologist in the world. I was not the best at CT or MRI, but I would match my skills in ultrasound and especially in my specific areas of expertise to be among the best in the world. With diligent consistent focus in one specific area you enjoy, you can't help but get good. You cannot possibly be the absolute best at everything, but you can be *the absolute best* at one thing.

What one *specific* problem can you solve, that you want to solve and that you have a track record in solving for at least yourself or someone else? You will get bonus points if people are already coming to you for advice in this area. That is going to make your life a lot easier if they are already seeking you out. Many times, it is hard for us to see our own zone of genius. It is sometimes so natural for us that we discount it and don't see the value in it. It is like the niche is so close to us and such a part of us—like right behind our ear—that we can't even see it. Sometimes we think that everyone knows what we know or thinks like we think. Sometimes it is useful to think of how you are different from others to help differentiate you from others. Even start very general and then incrementally become more specific. For example, if someone is sick, my husband may feel bad for them, but he has no urge to rush out and help them heal like I do. On the other hand, if he sees a car that is damaged, he feels an urge to fix it and rehabilitate it. I, on the other hand, could care less. I might have a preference for cars to be taken care of and look nice, but I am not losing any sleep over it. So, this gets us started in the very broad categories of health versus cars for example. From there, let's spiral in further to create that very specific niche that will be the one doorway for your clients to find you in the noisy jungle.

So, considering what you want from Chapter 3 and pairing it with the specific problem you want to and can solve, write down what that is. Now I can almost guarantee you it is way too general. Every one of my clients starts with their *specific* problem and posts it in our group only to realize it is actually several problems or really vague in "coach speak" and not in the language of their ideal client. So, your ideal client is not going to be able to hear, see or find you. But this is a great place to start. Just like cars versus health. Then move to a more specific health issue like weight loss, eating healthy or inflammation. Then make that more specific like thirty-pound weight loss or eating with allergies or rheumatoid arthritis. Then make that more specific like thirty-pound weight loss in a postpartum or a postmenopausal woman. You can see how even thirty-pound weight loss will be approached differently in a postpartum versus a postmenopausal woman and how your language and where you will find them is different. It is not actually the same specific problem although there will be certainly overlap in your approach.

If we take eating with allergies, we could do that for kids in a school program or teachers or moms or alternatively, we could focus on adults wanting to alleviate their own symptoms. Each of these as an ideal client is very different and the approach is going to be different and your ideal client might not actually be the one directly with the health concern. For example, your client could be the school board or a corporation and the specific problem from their perspective is going to be different than that of a mother of a child with allergies. The key is to know and be super specific as to whom you are serving and what specific aspect of the problem you are solving with your specific approach. If we look at the rheumatoid arthritis example, how old is your ideal client and what specifically is the problem? Lots of people help people with arthritis. How and for whom, are you the best in the world? Is it child athletes? Is it an elderly woman who lives alone who can't open her food containers or put on clothing? Or could it be for someone like my former dentist, who was highly skilled—a beautiful, intelligent, excellent dentist— forced to quit the career she had invested time and money in, because of her rheumatoid arthritis? Do you see how much more powerful your solution is for that one specific person—the dentist Dr. D.?

This is the secret sauce that most coaches miss. In their attempt to reach everyone, they reach no one. If you speak specifically to Dr. D., she will hear you. If this is actually a problem you can and want to solve, she will love you! She will invest in this solution from you the expert on your way to becoming world class! But she won't find you in the noisy jungle of ads for rheumatoid arthritis. She probably feels like she has been there, done that when she hears the generic ads. But in speaking directly to Dr. D., not only will she hear you but so will dental hygienists with arthritis and the husband of a dentist who happens to have arthritis and so on. They will start to try and fit you and your world-class program, rather than you trying to change your program to be the flavor of the month depending on who is in front of you and what their problem is.

When I created a beta program to help health coaches create their own signature wellness program in twelve weeks, the ideal client I was speaking to was specifically forty-five-year-old Dr. Ava Lynne, a character I created based on my former self and health coaching clients. Dr. Ava's specific problem was "How do I leave my lucrative medical career and still make a living healing?" This was a problem I had solved for myself and that I had health coaches and other health professionals asking me to solve and that I felt passionate about because I saw such a huge need.

This first program was filled in less than a week of conceiving the idea *and* the first three clients *came to me* before I had even breathed a word of it to anyone! They tried to fit my program. I would hear them say at the doorway to my specific program that they could find: "I'm a chiropractor not a medical doctor, can I come in?" "I'm a nurse and health coach, can I come in?" "I am younger than the others can I come in?" "I am a man, can I come in?" By being super specific about who I was creating this program for I quickly had it filled with ideal clients who I absolutely adored in under a week. Their questions about being allowed in were valid. My program isn't for everyone and we had an interview first to see if we would be a fit to work together further or not. I do not offer my program to all those I speak to either. I now only help people who want to be helped. Your clients' results, your word-of-mouth referrals, and satisfaction are greatly increased by selecting only those that are a fit for your program. But of those who want to be helped, by speaking to one specific person, many others can find the doorway to you and your program. Speak to one and you get to serve many.

This is so counter intuitive for most healers. They want to heal everyone but end up having no clients and healing no one. But this step is powerful. I have many great examples of how you help many by speaking to one. One of my awesome, coachable clients Jill was helping people with many health conditions including arthritis and autoimmune diseases. I continued to encourage her to get more and more specific. Given her amazing track record with her mom's rheumatoid arthritis and her passion and competence in this area, we decided this would be an excellent niche in which she could be world class. Somewhat disbelieving she told a referring functional medicine doctor that she was now specializing her practice to focus on patients with rheumatoid arthritis. Two days later this doctor called her and said, "I know you are only taking rheumatoid patients, but I have a client with autoimmune disease, and I was wondering if I could refer her to you?" Essentially, this doctor was trying to fit Jill's signature program. The way Jill was able to attract the autoimmune client (which she also could help) was to focus as an expert in rheumatoid. This is how you have people begging to work with you. This is how you fish and not hunt. Your specific niche is attractive "bait" and is infinitely more effective than chasing people—anyone with any problems—into the jungle when you hunt generically.

The critically important exercise in this chapter is to determine which *one person* with which *one specific problem* do you want to serve and what is the *one specific solution* you can deliver that you have a track record in and that you want to focus on to become world class? Grab your notebook. Write down the one person that is your ideal client. That is singular. Not clients. Who is your best client you want to serve? Who do you have a soul contract to work with? Write her bio or personal diary entry and include the following:

1. What is her/his name and specific age (not an age range)?
2. What does she do for a living?
3. Where does she live?
4. What is her specific problem that you could solve?
5. What would be her absolute best solution?
6. Why is this important for her to solve now?

Get in her head. Your success as a health coach is directly proportional to your ability to get super specific about your ideal client and their *one* problem that you can solve with a specific tangible result in language that an eight-year-old could understand. For example, their specific problem is what they are googling late at night trying to solve. It is "how do I lose weight?" It is not "how do I find myself?" If they know they are gluten intolerant, it might be "what foods are gluten-free and where can I find them?" It is not "how can I feel connected?" or "how can I love myself more?" Now almost certainly your program will show your client how to love herself (the solution to almost every problem) and feel more connected and "find herself" but she isn't actively looking for that. So, figure out what she is looking for that you can help with and then give her that but also what she *really* needs. For years my focus was healthy weight loss for a forty-year-old busy mom. I helped a lot more than one busy forty-year-old woman named Ava with weight loss. In fact, I helped thousands of men and women with weight loss. But by speaking to one person, people could hear me and know how I could help them. This was a specific problem I could solve that they were already looking for and asking for my help with and was a problem I had already solved for myself. What they received was so much more than weight loss. I believe there is a saying "sell them what they want, give them what they (really) need."

Your ideal client can be your former self or modelled after one of your clients or a composite of clients. But give her a specific name other than yours. Everything that follows hinges on you knowing who this person is. You will almost certainly not be specific enough in your first attempt. That's okay. Keep at it. Keep going until you know what she ate for breakfast and what she thought about last night before bed.

So again, get crystal clear on the *one person* you want to serve and which *one specific problem* you can solve with which one *specific solution* that you have a track record in and that you want to focus on to become world class. The focus on *one* is how you serve many. Even as you begin to focus on this one person now, watch for them to begin to show up in your experience. It will start to feel like magic or maybe that there are surveillance cameras on your journal entries. It will defy logic but that is how you will know you are really onto something and aligned with your soul's purpose. This happens all the time for myself and my clients. In the next chapter we will focus on how to best deliver this world-class solution for you and your ideal client.

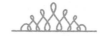

Chapter 5

Align Your Program to
Be the Best Solution

"A person who sees a problem is a human being; a person who finds a solution is a visionary; and the person who goes out and does something about it is an entrepreneur."

–Naveen Jain

With clarity on what you want and who you can serve and what specific problem you can solve, the next question is how can you best serve your ideal client? There are many ways to serve but what I am going to show you is how to create a soul-satisfying signature program that is the best solution for your client and yourself as well as some of the pitfalls to avoid and some early steps to take.

In the last chapter, I emphasized (or, more accurately, hammered home) the importance of picking a specific problem. This allows your client to get results and find you, but also is helpful to create a program that clearly addresses something specific. This allows you to build one business that solves one problem for one person and scale from there. This allows you to become world class. Now the nature of your ideal client's problem is going to influence the best particular solution for you. But here are some options to consider:

1. Live versus online
2. Group versus one-on-one
3. Speaking to large audiences versus smaller workshops
4. Individual personal clients versus corporate wellness programs
5. Retreats
6. VIP days versus monthly or three- or six-month or year-long commitments

There is definitely more than one right answer, but some options suit your personality and your client's personality and needs better than others. You can do a combination but don't do all of them (at least not all right away) and again the more you can simplify this the better.

All methods have their unique benefits. For example, when I first began coaching over a decade ago, I met clients in my sun room that looked out over the river. It was lovely. I had spa music playing. A fresh pot of green tea was enjoyed. My clients felt warm, invited, and relaxed and it was enjoyable for me, too. I met my clients mainly individually or in couples and they got amazing results and it was a wonderful learning experience for me to see their transformations and learn what things worked best. I liked being able to sit in silence and not always jump in to answer for them. I liked to be able to read their body language and give them a hug. The disadvantages were that I had to make sure that my kids and dog were not home or making noise. I always prepped ahead, making the green tea, getting the environment ready, and cleaning the house. Plus, our appointments were supposed to be one hour, but I almost always went over. I really enjoyed seeing my clients, and I believe they really enjoyed seeing me, too. Having them in my home where I also entertained friends with no time limits led to a blurred boundary with not always an absolute cut-off time. In the early days there wasn't always a client waiting right after. There was no receptionist to keep our schedule. Many of these disadvantages can be easily corrected and this option works for some people.

I also tried meeting my clients publicly at a coffee shop or restaurant. The downside of this was I always felt rushed driving through traffic to get there on time. There was, of course, the added expense of whatever we bought; more importantly, we often discussed very sensitive issues that they couldn't share with anyone else in detail, and a public place was not the best. Plus, I could not stack clients back-to-back. It proved to be a very inefficient way for me to connect with my clients. However, if you have a gym, spa, or wellness center or doctor's office where you can connect with clients, then many of the disadvantages above are solved. If you only need to go to one workplace and especially if that is where your clients are hanging out anyways, this can be a great option.

For years now, I have met my clients over the phone. I love that my morning commute from the bedroom to the boardroom is about five seconds. I love that I can wear my yoga pants. I love that my family is not disturbed by me and vice versa. I love that I can stack appointments back-to-back on a schedule that I determine. I actually like the phone appointments for my clients too. They don't have to drive to me or get ready to see me. In fact, the vast majority of my clients are not local. About half don't even live in the same country. I can take notes readily while my clients are talking and without the visual, my ability to listen is sharpened in a different way—hearing what is meant beyond what is said.

Your best program to deliver your best solution may also depend on whether your program delivers something physical that requires your live presence or whether your clients are local or global. The online option should not be dismissed too readily as impersonal, however. This is a common misconception amongst new health coaches or with healers such as doctors or nurses used to seeing their patients face to face. There are many ways to create a great personal and effective program where you can still see and talk with each other live even though you are not physically in the same room.

Another factor to consider is whether you want to coach individuals or groups. As a medical doctor I was used to seeing patients one at a time. In the beginning as a health coach, I mainly saw clients individually although I used to give talks to larger groups or a series of talks to focused groups. I used to think that groups were just a cheaper alternative for people who couldn't afford private coaching or for people early in their journey who weren't as committed to getting results. While all of this could be the case, I learned that was not nearly always the case. After being in high-level mastermind groups as a participant and also as a coach of high-level groups there is the potential for even greater value with the group dynamic. For example, as I coach a small group of nine people to create their signature wellness programs in twelve weeks, answering one person's question can almost always benefit the rest. They may not yet have even formulated that question themselves. Often people can hear the answer better in the answer to someone else when they aren't in their head about what they are going to say next or when the subject matter isn't something so personal to which they are attached. I similarly have participated in groups where I can understand the mentor's teachings better as it is demonstrated over and over with multiple examples. I then notice that if I believe the mentor is correct with all these other participants, that the chance of me being the one exception to their advice is highly unlikely and that makes me trust the process and surrender my attachments to old familiar ways that may not be serving me. In an effective group, there is a natural accountability process that develops too and that can inspire success. As you see other mere mortals just like you become successful, you are apt to think if they can do it, so can you. If everyone else has done their homework, you feel you better get on this in a positive peer pressure way.

There are a few common pitfalls to consider when creating your signature program. For example, being too general is the most common one and we really addressed that in the last chapter. Make sure you are delivering a solution to one specific problem with a tangible specific result. Often health and well-being can be vague and encompass many factors, so how do you make it specific? Focusing on that one aspect of it for one specific person that you can be world class in is a great start and then adding a time frame or some other specificity to it also helps. Consider the example from the previous chapter of a postpartum mom wanting to lose thirty pounds. If your program delivers that solution in three months, it becomes much more likely that she will find you and join your program than if you just said I help people lose weight. The actual amount of time isn't the important part and will vary depending on the problem you solve but people like to know there is a specific start and stop to this and that at the end of your program they will have the specific result.

When choosing time frames for your program, sometimes the options are obvious as in a one-day VIP day or a three-day retreat. But your time frame options are broader when you are creating your program to coach your clients through to a solution in a more traditional coaching program. Six months is a popular traditional time frame being long enough to change habits and get results and not so short that you are always needing to get new clients or feel like you are always asking your existing clients for more money. But it is also not years long or an undetermined duration. Six months is what I was trained to do and did do initially for years and can be a great option. Year-long programs can work great for very specific committed high-level individual clients but not generally as great for the masses. However, a year-long program could work well if you are coaching individuals or a small group through to 100-pound weight loss whereas a thirty-day program wouldn't make sense.

In more recent years, a lot of my programs have been thirty to ninety days. People are great at focusing for thirty days. Beyond ninety days though they often require re-invigoration. People don't like to get "locked in" to something for too long and they also want to see specific results right away. Their attention spans seem shorter than they were a decade ago. People are used to living in trimesters. Pregnancies and seasons naturally change in trimesters or every ninety days. Business tracking is also divided into ninety-day quarters of the year. Life generally changes with the seasons in what people do and aligning your program with this can support your success.

The next pitfall is getting trapped into trading time for money. Most coaches often start off charging an hourly rate. They may charge a monthly rate with a fixed number of sessions each month, but it is essentially time for money. This is an okay place to start and is where I started but there are two fundamental issues with this. First, people aren't really wanting to pay to talk to you. Instead what they want to pay for is a specific result which is why you want to have your program set up to deliver a specific result. Often a faster result is even more valuable. The other issue you will quickly realize is that there are only so many hours in a month. This means there is a limit on your income. This can prevent healers from doing their soul-satisfying work as their sole income. Unable to leave their day job, their health coaching practice often gets relegated to a hobby or more often than not, sacrificed completely so that they can still enjoy their family in their off time rather than spend years trying to get a second business off the ground that just doesn't have traction.

Let's play with some numbers to demonstrate this. Let's say that you charge $1,000 for your six-month program. For an annual income of $60,000 you would serve sixty clients. That could be thirty clients in each half of the year. Let's say you see them every other week for one hour, that would mean you see fifteen clients each week. That sounds pretty doable and it can be although most people already have another existing career when they start so they are trying to fit these fifteen hours into their "spare" time. Plus, there is the additional time required to attract these sixty new clients each year and interview them, etc. It is definitely doable but also a lot harder while you are working another career and you can do both for a little while but eventually most people feel they have to pick one like I did. Going in two directions forever just isn't sustainable. (This is when a lot of coaches reach out to me for guidance because they see that I did this, while most people aren't able to create a health coaching career that makes a living and a difference.)

The other aspect is holding the space for thirty clients at a time to create their transformations is a lot! And while $60,000 may be something that allows some to make a great living, it certainly is not enough to replace a medical career and all of the monthly expenses that non-medical people don't realize you have. I know at one point my college dues, insurance, licensing and corporation fees and just basic food and housing (no vacations, eating out, clothing, entertainment nor savings) was $11,000 a month in expenses. So, filling every waking minute catering to these clients and all the website and marketing involved was not even going to come close to covering my expenses even if I found a way to cut back on my medical career. My medical income could go down, but my fixed expenses did not. If I tried to double my coaching practice to double my income so that I could get myself to barely break even (and cut my overall income severely in the process) so I could at least remotely consider leaving my medical career, the numbers still didn't add up. Now to fit in 120 clients per year or sixty clients every six months or thirty clients each week (and sixty clients' stories and journeys to hold the space for at a time)…that is thirty extra hours each week to fit in my "spare" time of which I had none. If I thought I was burned out before…!

This becomes the trap that many highly talented health professionals find themselves in and they never do break free and end up giving up on their dreams and their soul-satisfying work to continue to fall back on their day job, pushing out their happiness until a someday that never comes. By that I mean happiness is not something that occurs in the future. It is now o'clock. If we'll be happy when…we actually won't ever be happy (more on this in Chapter 7). Now, don't get me wrong, if people are highly satisfied in their medical careers, that is fantastic. Keep going! You probably aren't reading this book. But if your actual calling and desire for your life has you interested in this book, then don't despair. I will show you the way. But I wanted to point out the actual pitfalls that health coaches fall into along their journey and how to overcome them.

So, it is possible that you have someone else paying your bills and your income is a bonus and that $60,000 to $120,000 is a fantastic income and at fifteen to thirty hours a week, working from home is a dream come true and that you can easily fit in at least a weekly full administrative day and a self-care day to keep this sustainable.

But if you have another full-time job or you are the sole bread winner or you require more to make your ends meet, then listen up! One of the best ways I found to serve my clients was through online courses. I could give my very best information through videos on a particular subject via several modules that I created to walk my clients through the steps to get their desired result. They could watch the information at their convenience in their time zone as many times as they wanted. Then to be sure that they had their individual questions answered and they were supported, the program also included a specific Facebook group. In the group, supplemental and new information could be delivered and each week I had a specific Q&A live video call where we could see and converse with each other so that they could get their very best results.

This worked extremely well and although I spent many hours creating the modules and delivering world-class content, once it was created, it was created. Now my work was condensed to that one hour a week Q&A call. The clients got great value! They got actual specific tangible results from a specific program and also my undivided attention on those calls. All of their questions were answered in the group that I was active in each day. It was a win-win. I had a four-step game plan that I followed and then taught in a program I developed to teach health coaches to do the same. In the *30-Day Course Creator*, I teach health coaches how to create their own online courses and how to attract and support their clients through the entire process.

Online education is the way of the future. Think about it. When you have a problem or question, what do you do? You google it. This is where people are going for answers. Online education is a $100 billion-dollar industry. I guarantee there are things you know that other people want to know. Online courses allow you to share transformational impactful information to a larger audience and automate it. So, you do the work once—*your* work in your soul-satisfying niche—once and you can create impact repeatedly and income repeatedly ... even while you sleep or spend time with your family! It is a fantastic way to duplicate yourself. I cannot tell you how incredible it is to do amazing work and teach your area of expertise and then while you are at a movie with your spouse or sleeping, someone from half way across the world enrolls in your online program on their journey to get amazing results!

That is my favorite way to get around the pitfall of trading time for money and give you time freedom, location freedom and create soul-satisfying work that makes a difference in a highly scalable way! I am so passionate about this aspect that I include my teaching of this, giving lifetime access to the twelve modules of the *30-Day Course Creator*, to all of my clients that are creating their own signature programs.

Of course, there are other ways to get around the trading time for money ceiling and that would include other income sources from other products that may be aligned with your specific niche such as nutritional supplements, essential oils, skin care products, etc. But focus is always important in being successful at anything and I remember hearing someone at a lecture once say that *Focus* stands for Follow One Course Until Successful. I agree with this. Plus, it is extremely challenging to build multiple businesses and some companies may have rules about this. Ideally you want that *one* specific doorway to your program for your clients to find you in the noisy jungle. Adding multiple products as upfront offers creates a very noisy jungle and a very confusing message and it is not clear at all what you specifically do. Pick one problem and one solution in which to become world class and in your toolkit once people are in your program, there may be additional items that you wholeheartedly believe are the absolute best to deliver the best results for your clients that you may want to include. The one nice thing about having your own signature program is that it is yours. No one can take that away from you and you are truly your own boss.

Sometimes people shy away from the online approach because it sounds impersonal. Let me share with you one option that can give you the best of both worlds. You could create the core information that you teach to everyone in an online course. Then weekly you could offer group or individual coaching to members in your program that gives that highly personal aspect that helps ensure your clients are on track and get their best results.

The last few pitfalls fall under the category of starting too big, judging too early and switching too soon. Sometimes people hear of coaches having seven figure businesses and they want that right away or I heard someone last week at a conference say that she wanted to heal fifty million people and get funding to pay for that so the clients wouldn't have to pay for it themselves. You just know that is never ever going to happen—not in any fantasy world. Now on the other hand if she focused on one person to help and achieve excellent results and charged her client just a little or even free for that first client as she is learning herself; then from that result attract another client and then another. So that one client becomes two and then three and five and ten and thirty and then she would also raise her rates with her experience. That is the way to have a successful business that can then fund her movement that she can become world class in and scale, and then she can do pro bono work, and create a foundation, and perhaps even serve millions. But the key is to start small. It has to be believable to you for it to work. You can easily psyche yourself out if you have too grandiose of a goal. You can have a vision to climb a huge mountain. You can want to climb Mount Everest but let's start by then focusing on the first base camp that you can see and is believable and is within reach, and that we can take the baby steps toward. That works!

When we start with a huge goal that can lead us to judge ourselves as a failure too early. We may not know how to reach the top of the mountain and we stop before we get started. We get stuck in the overwhelm, doubt, frustrated side of our map. We want to be on the belief and optimistic side of the map. If someone wants to lose 100 pounds and in the first two weeks they only lose one pound, they can judge themselves a failure and quit too soon. If you are trying to create your program, and you have done the exercises in the previous chapter, and you know your ideal client with their specific problem and solution, and then before you even test it out, you start to think too big, and then judge it as not working because you aren't there yet—you may be tempted to switch to another idea or another program. You can keep chasing shiny objects and never get your program launched. The key again is *positive focus, taking baby steps, in the direction that you want.* Give it your absolute focus and don't change direction until you have proven to yourself that it needs to be adjusted and we will talk about that in the next chapter.

For now, here are some baby steps you can take today. Now that you know who your ideal client is, what is the best format for you and them? If you have absolutely no idea what type of program to start creating, keep it simple. Start with individual clients in a three-month coaching program that delivers a specific solution to their specific problem via weekly one-hour phone appointments.

Next, start to attract and gather your tribe. Where do your ideal clients hang out? For my client Tim who helps single dads who are pre-diabetic looking to get back in shape and be a great role model for their kids, that is at the gym. For my client Val who helps Christian empty-nest moms reignite the spark in their marriage, there are Christian women support and fellowship groups. For my client Jill who helps women with rheumatoid arthritis, there is a functional medicine doctor who is a referral source for her and rheumatologists. For my client Nicole who helps women post bariatric surgery, there are bariatric surgeons' offices and online support groups. For my client Jennifer who helps women with polycystic ovaries, that is online support groups, gynecologists' offices and even an ultrasound clinic where they are diagnosed. The more specific you are about who you serve, the easier it is to pinpoint where you can find them. But also, to the extent that you are willing to work *with* doctors rather than against them, respecting each of your roles, this can open up a great referral source for you.

Once you know where they gather physically or virtually in various support groups etc., how can you position yourself in front of them? You may even just stumble upon this too. For Tim it happened to be in the steam room at the gym where the conversation inevitably turned to health and he could clearly state what he did. This led to booked appointments to find out more. For many of you it could be free or paid talks to your group—either live or virtually. This is how my client attracted in one week nine clients into her ten-week program from a live workshop (which also earned her over $10,000 and she is worth every penny!). This is how I built my practice. I did many health talks at businesses, in schools, to teachers, at the hospital, as part of health curriculums in the community, to women's groups and these were primarily to forty-year-old busy working moms. Nowadays, free private Facebook groups are a great way to teach on your niche to people who are wanting that information, and this is now my primary way to attract and serve my following.

So, write down in your notebook what you believe is the best way to align your program to be the best solution for your client and you. Then write down where does your ideal client hang out and how you could connect with them. Is it live conversation like Tim? Is it with a brochure to patients like Jill and Jennifer? Is it a live community talk like Catherine? Is it a blog or podcast? Is it via Facebook groups like myself? I really like the Facebook option currently. It is my single most successful option. In fact, what I recommend as you move throughout your day and meet people you enjoy and connect with is to Facebook friend them just to stay connected. No agenda. I realized that of the clients in my initial beta group, I only knew two of them the year prior but all of them had become my Facebook friends sometime in the past year, allowing us a convenient way to stay in touch. Make that a habit to pull out your phone when you meet someone wonderful and ask them if they are on Facebook, and then find them right then and there, and send them a request. They can choose to accept or not. Don't pitch. Never pitch. As one of my mentors says, "The prize never chases." Just stay in touch. And if they happen to resonate with your messaging, they will be drawn in the most wonderful way to you allowing you to fill your soul-satisfying signature program with ease in an organic way. In the next chapter, we will take the next steps to refine what you do and how you do it even further.

Chapter 6

Keep Inching Forward with Baby Steps

"If one advances confidently in the direction of his dreams and endeavors to live the life which he has imagined, he will meet with a success unexpected in common hours."
–Henry David Thoreau

Now that we are gaining increasing clarity on what we want, who we serve, and how we serve them, the next step is to inch forward and test the waters before we actually invest thousands of hours and dollars in creating websites and modules and branding. What we want to know is whether you have actually created a visible doorway that your ideal clients can find in the jungle. Does your ideal client actually word their problem in the same language as you do? Can they clearly understand who you are and what you do and specifically how you can deliver their dream come true? Is this a problem they are actively looking to solve and willing to invest in themselves to solve? If they are not, it is a lot better to find that out now before you get too attached to your beautiful expensive and time-consuming website or program. This is a common mistake many new health coaches make. Working on websites "seems" like they are working on their business. A clever excuse to hide out that those around you will often support. Far better to actually help a human however, and then once you have a growing clientele, create a website that conveys your message and indicates you are legit. (Fun fact: I have never gotten a client because of my website. I may have sent them there, but even the best website is not actually an awareness campaign).

The absolute best way to test out what you have to offer is… to offer it! Doing an offer to your beta program under construction is the best win-win for you and them. They get valuable results at a discounted price. They tend to get a lot of your undivided attention as their success is your success. This is a great way to test out how clear and specific you have been with your messaging. This is where you will learn that if you chose to stay vague, you now have no idea where to find women who want to "find themselves" and even if you do amongst some friends, none of them are actually willing to invest in you to solve that problem. However, if you chose to focus specifically on thirty-pound weight loss in a postpartum mom in your twelve-week program where she will lose her baby weight before she goes back to work so she doesn't need a whole new office wardrobe… you know exactly where to find her in mom's groups. These women often hang out together on playdates. Word of mouth referrals spread like wildfire! As one woman in the group gets her body back, the others will come to *you* without you even having to ask! Now in your program, you can help these women find themselves in their new role and identity as mom and what that means to who she really is. But what they are initially after is to fit back in their jeans and get a bit of their sexy back. There are other successful specific niches beyond weight loss, that is just the one I used for years to teach people about self-care and clean eating and even their soul's purpose—so that is the one I have the most examples to reference. It is important to understand what your ideal client is looking for at the moment. Some health issues actually become trendy. As people become educated and aware, specific health issues can become buzz words that people are actively wanting to understand. My client Rachel serves the common busy mom demographic expertly, by adding her focus on gut health. Gut health is not a gimmick and it is an essential component of Rachel's signature program, but it is also something that her clients are wanting now, whereas they may not have been searching for this ten years ago. But regardless of your niche, if you are very specific, that helps you to know where to find your ideal client, what message resonates with them and even what to include in your program to deliver the absolute best results.

The first baby step in creating your beta offer is to get crystal clear on what you do in one sentence. Otherwise known sometimes as an elevator pitch, this power statement is something that is great to have just roll off your tongue. It is not a paragraph that feels salesy. It is not your list of accomplishments or how great you are. It is a casual one-liner that indicates *when asked* what you actually do and for whom, without you rambling all over the place and having you look like someone who is trying to find herself (cue the quirky emoji). I am sure you have all been at parties where someone is going on and on about what they do, and you have zero interest and you're not remotely their ideal client and you are just looking for a polite way to exit. Don't be that person. I am going to teach you a way to attract not push away your ideal client—how to fish not hunt.

But first let's answer "what do you do?" We are going to piece together your work from the previous chapters into one power statement following a specific formula that looks something like this in language an eight-year-old could understand:

"I help (ideal client) with (specific problem) to (specific result) in (timeframe) so they can (bonus benefit)."

Here is an example when asked what you do:

"I help (new moms) who (are struggling to lose that baby fat) (get back to their pre-pregnancy weight) in (three months) so they can (get back in their skinny jeans, feel great, and be a great role model for their kids)."

The specifics obviously depend on what you do, and you can omit the timeframe component if this is a casual conversation. But it is pretty clear whether your program is for them or not. It is very clear on what you do. That is extremely attractive, and you can say that with clarity and confidence.

Contrast the above example with this alternative answer:

"I used to be a nurse and then I became a health coach because I like helping people and I can really help people with their health so much more now and the schedule is a much better fit for me. I show people what to eat so they can be healthy and get results. We do meditation and I also teach yoga and I do acupuncture and reiki and massage, and I really like helping people find out who they really are."

Do you have any idea how this person could actually help you? When could you expect what results? Or how you would actually work together? This is how coaches hide in the jungle. This statement screams, "I mean well but I am finding myself right now and trying to figure out what I am doing with my life. Want me to help you figure out what to do with your life?"

Another important point here is that people don't really care about how you do it. They may say they do and as coaches we very much care about our process, *but* your prospective clients do not, and this is a trap where you can lose them. If you confuse them, you lose them. You can't possibly share everything that you do with someone to get their results in one conversation. But if you share a little bit of your process, they might think they can do it on their own and they don't know what they don't know. Or they may think they have tried that before or know someone else who has tried that before and dismiss you. But the truth is they have never done your world-class program with *you*. So, the best thing you can do for your prospective clients is speak clearly and confidently about the specific problem and the specific solution you deliver and for whom. That's it.

After that one-line power statement and to avoid the sometimes-awkward silence that follows and to prevent it from sounding like a pitch, I will immediately add the following question: "How about you? What do you do?" So, for example, this could look like:

"I help pre-diabetic single dads who want to lose weight and balance their blood sugars to lose fifty pounds in six months so they can be a great living role model for their kids. *How about you? What do you do?*"

Again, you could omit the specific "fifty pounds in six months" if this is a casual conversation. Now as they are answering that question, they will be thinking about what you just said, and you may have peaked their curiosity which is the point. They may come back to you then or even months later, trying to fit themselves or someone they know into your program instead of the other way around. They may say "I'm not a single dad. I'm a single mom. Can I come in?" "I'm not pre-diabetic but I want to lose weight. Can I come in?" "I don't have kids and I only have ten pounds to lose. Can I come in?" You now have a clear doorway to invite people into your program and you get to decide if you want to invite them inside.

Now if you are having this conversation and you already know what they do for a living then you could say something else to divert the conversation back to them. Something like "How about your business? How long have you been doing that?" or "How about you? What is new with you?"

Then in a cocktail party or networking scenario, wait for *them* to ask you for more details. Remember, we are fishing not hunting. You don't want to chase and scare them off into the jungle. You just dangle the bait which is you. If they don't ask, they aren't interested. Leave them alone. You have clearly stated what you do and for whom. There is no need to give more if they are not asking. If they are asking for details, then be a professional. Let them know you would be happy to do that but now is not really the place where you can give them your undivided attention, so set up an appointment within the week. Ideally set the appointment the next day while they still are remotely curious. Set a firm date and time when they can give you their undivided attention and write it down and send an appointment reminder. Be a professional. This already will start to inspire within them confidence that you are the leader they want to follow in your program that will deliver results. Regardless, you can strengthen that connection by sending them a Facebook friend request like I mentioned previously. Instead of waiting until you get home or the next day, when it may look like you are stalking them, ask them if they are on Facebook and pull your phone out in the moment. Say something like you'd love to stay connected. Then hand them your phone and say, "Find yourself." Then you can click the friend request. The option to accept is still totally up to them and they can do that later. So often though I can't find the actual person I spoke to later on Facebook given multiple people with the same name. This is just such an excellent way to stay in touch and now the majority of my clients come from this little practice and sometimes not even for months or years later when their time is right for what I offer. This practice is a great way to organically grow your tribe.

At the appointment, you will find out about them and what they are looking for. You will see what they have tried before and how important it is for them to solve this problem right now. You will find out why they want their result, what it is costing them not to solve the result and their commitment level to solving it. Perhaps they were just being polite and don't really have the problem or they don't really want to solve the problem, or their problem is not something that you can solve. Essentially you are determining if you are a fit to work together or not. At the beginning of your coaching career you may be tempted to help anyone with a pulse and a credit card, but this is a really bad idea for both of you. If people don't really want to solve the problem and if you want the results more than they do, you are going to be pulling your hair out and be exhausted and you will question your program when it is just not a right fit for them. Some people would literally rather die than change and they have that right. You wouldn't want them to force their lifestyle on you, so don't force your clean eating healthy lifestyle on them. Help only those who want to be helped. A burning desire to have their problem solved should be a characteristic of your ideal client.

Then if they are a fit, you can ask if they have questions for you and again wait for them to ask about your program. You can state your one-liner power statement of "what you do" again to refresh their memory but for everything else, let them ask you. If they are not asking, they aren't interested. If they are, you can let them know initially that you are doing a new beta program. Beta by the way doesn't mean experimenting to see if you can solve the problem. The problem that you solve is a problem that you know you *can* and *want* to solve. The beta program is the first iteration of your signature program as a new way of delivering your expertise. So, it may be adding on an online component such as an online course or private FB group. It may be while a new branding process is underway with your new website that will be updated, and you are gathering additional success stories perhaps. Or it can be honestly that you are just starting out but that you have solved this problem for yourself and then a handful of others who've asked you (the reluctant hero). Now you are looking to give structure and organization to your proven process.

So perfect. You now know exactly what to say when someone asks you "What do you do?" But how do you get someone to ask that? Well there is a natural law of reciprocity. If someone asks you, "How are you?" the natural tendency is to reply, "I'm fine. How are you?" So, if you would like someone to ask you what you do, ask them what they do! Or if you already know that, you can ask them about their business or what's new. This is normal chatter at parties and events. With a slight twist as in "What have you been up to lately?" at the office water cooler, you may get the same question back and away you go.

But what if you don't see people in these scenarios? Well, start to attend events live or virtually where your ideal clients hang out. Again, another reason it is important to know who and where they are. If you are wanting to reach busy women that is still general but if you narrow it down to military wives or oil wives like my client Lana, now you know their specific issues and the language they use and where they hang out. This doesn't have to be super formal. For example, you can be talking with another mom watching your children on the playground and in conversation, you can ask if they are planning to stay home with their new baby or if they are going back to a workplace. They will in turn ask you. It is very common for any conversation in any niche to turn to health. You could even interject if appropriate with a "That's very interesting. That is actually what I do. I help…"

Your goal here is eventually to make the offer to your beta program but you are going to do that in a specific order that maintains relationships and only gives information to those people that are asking. This can be summarized as follows:

1. *Connect* over something that you share in common that forms a connection.
2. *Share* what you do in one power statement sentence *if they ask*.
3. *Invite* them to book an appointment *if they ask for details.*
4. *Offer* your beta program *if they are a fit for your program.*

You can also do this virtually via Facebook or over the phone or via videos. This may be very similar to what I have outlined above but sometimes it is more of a one-way communication as in a Facebook live video. In this case, still connect but get straight to the point. So, your video could be something like this:

"Hey friends! Hope you are having a fabulous day! I am super excited to share something with you that I am starting next week. It is definitely not for everyone and in fact it can only be for a few of you given the nature of it, but I thought I would ask here in case this would be a dream come true for you. Some of you know that I have been helping people with their health but specifically what I do is—I help (ideal client) with (specific problem) to get (specific result) in (timeframe) so they can (bonus benefit). So, I am starting this fantastic program next week. If you are a (ideal client) that wants (result) in the next (timeframe), message me and we can set up an appointment to find out more about your situation to see if this program would be a fit for you or not. If it sounds like this might be for you then fantastic, I would love to talk to you. If not, that is cool too and regardless I wish you all a fantastic day. Cheers!"

That is it. Super simple. Gets straight to the point. No convincing or arm twisting. Takes less than sixty seconds to say. Be professional. No laundry hanging in the background. Sit up straight or stand. Then from the messages that you get, send them a link to book a time on your calendar. This is why I like using calendar software to save time with this but at the beginning you can message back and forth to set a time that works for you. But very quickly I believe it is worth investing a little bit to have scheduling software so you can send them a link to your available times, and they can easily book a time that works for them. This software usually sends out appointment reminders which is great.

Now, the next critical thing is *do not answer any questions through text or message!* If you answer one, you will be typing all day and they will never book a time and you will never find out about them and they will never be your client. You cannot give a price because you do not know if they are a fit for your program or not. If they are not willing to get on the phone for a free appointment that will ultimately lead to their problem solved, they are not coachable, and they are not likely to really want to invest the time and energy to solve the problem. Just let them go. Let them know you want to find out all about their particular situation to see if your program is something that would be of benefit or perhaps there is something else that would be better. If they ask what the price is right away that is almost an immediate disqualification for your program. If they won't get on the phone without this information, that is definitely an immediate disqualification because that question doesn't even make sense up front. Because a dollar amount without context is meaningless and if the value is great enough one could argue the cost doesn't really matter. If someone asked, "How much?" and I said $100. What does that mean? If it is $100 for a piece of paper, that is expensive! If it is for a Ferrari, that is a deal! Asking that question up front also implies that they aren't super committed to solving the problem yet.

When someone is what I call "high noon" and ripe and ready for change and they really want a particular result, the cost is not the prime concern but rather, they just want to know this will work. If it does, it will be worth it. Think back in your life when you invested but it was so worth it because you got exactly what you wanted. How awesome was that?! Now think back to times when you invested, and you did not get what you wanted. It was a waste of your time and money. How awful did that feel? So, it isn't really the cost that matters but rather whether your program delivers. This is why we want a specific result, so we know, and your clients know, that your world-class program delivers! If we help someone "find themselves" or "feel more connected," how do we know if that worked? On the other hand, if someone loses weight or has their blood sugar balanced or is able to cut back on pain or allergy medication, we can tell your program works! People buy results. Results make you feel great too because you have happy clients that love you for it!

So, solve problems you can solve and become world class at it. Word of mouth is still the best referral source for clients. This chapter has you taking that baby step to put yourself out there. Come from the love side of the map not fear. Focus in the positive direction and take those baby steps. Some people refer to this as failing forward. But essentially, we won't know if you are on track until you put the offer out there and see if your offer is bait that anyone wants or can see. If you have followed the steps so far this is likely going to be far easier than you could ever have imagined, and you may wonder why you were hiding so long in the jungle. Go for the micro wins because that is absolutely the secret of success!

An important but quick word on baby steps and micro wins. In 2009 and 2010, I had three close family members die suddenly with no warning within four months of each other in separate incidents. Specifically, in April 2010, my sister-in-law died suddenly in Alberta, and within twenty-four hours my mother-in-law died in

Manitoba. We were overwhelmed with grief. It just kept coming. I had already started to work as a health coach as well as a medical doctor and I was so frustrated that the people I cared about the most, I couldn't help. I was so stressed. My belly ballooned. I was totally off my game. I wondered why even bother to try and help people be healthy because we're just going to die anyway. I was really stuck in a dark place (and that comfort food is so not comforting). I knew that previously meditation, exercise and journaling had been really helpful for me, but I just couldn't do it. I totally didn't feel like it. I was stuck on the grief side of the map. But I decided one day to focus on what I *could do* rather than what I couldn't do. I couldn't do much but, what could I do? I could do one minute— sixty seconds of meditation and sixty seconds of exercise and sixty seconds of journaling. I could do one minute. And the next day I did two. And the next day I did three. And little by little I inched myself forward in the positive direction back to health, joy, and ease. If you need to set that bar really low to get a win—you do it! Just keep inching forward.

When my dad was in the hospital with his stroke, I wanted to keep us focused in the positive direction and on what was working when it felt like the rest of the world was focused on what wasn't working and in the opposite direction. So, I hung a calendar in my dad's room and each night I put a post-it note of our "win of the day." Things like: Off oxygen. IV out. Able to take sips. Able to wiggle finger. Able to lift leg. Able to stand (best day of my life that day!) Then steps. Cycling. Stairs. And these tiny little baby steps led him to walk out of the hospital on his own two feet in a record thirty-five days defying all the odds! Remember I shared previously that the day my dad went home from the hospital there was a woman half his age, with half as severe a stroke who was just starting to stand. This is the tremendous value of inching forward with baby steps.

As you start to put yourself out there, start small and keep focusing on what is working and ignore the rest. Keep focusing on what you can do (not on what you can't do). Help one person extremely well and find satisfaction in that and then scale from there. So, write out and practice your one power sentence. From a place of love and ease, invite people to an appointment following the guidelines in this chapter and let's make that offer to the beta version of your signature program to those ideal clients with a burning desire for you to help them solve their problem. Then start to write out and acknowledge your win of the day that will help keep you positively focused forward. In the next chapter, we are going to talk about elevating yourself to your soul's purpose (I'll let you in on a secret: this is my real reason for writing this book to share this life-changing information that you will love—while we give you what you want— your signature program). Onward and upward, my friends!

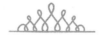

Chapter 7

Elevate Yourself to Your Soul's Purpose

"Let the natural flow of the universe course through your being and harmonize your soul."

–Ram Dass

I am so excited to share with you this next tool—*The BGOOD4U Awakening Elevator*™! This is my favorite tool that I use every day myself and teach to my clients—and they love it! I refined this tool after working with my dad and explaining the map to clients and then trying to teach people how to tap into their innate healing ability and heal themselves. So, if you recall from Chapter 3, when we discussed the map, at the top right corner we had point B which was what you really wanted and who you really are which is pure wellness. What we are going to do now is show you how you can use the elevator tool to lift you out of wherever you are to wherever you want to be. In other words, take you from the problem to the solution and from dis-ease to ease! *Because, as Einstein famously stated, "No problem can be solved from the same level of consciousness that created it."*

Most people get stuck in their problem, like I was stuck in my grief after my family passed or stuck in my struggle for years at the hospital. But the solution is not at the same level as the problem. It is not on the same side of the map. So, I found the visual of this elevator tool I created to be a great way to lift me up to where I wanted to be and to my soul's purpose and in turn, now to assist my clients to get to where they desire too. The general principles have been well known by many gurus over the years, but I decided to give it a practical tool application that we can put into practice. As Maharishi Mahesh Yogi stated, *"Analyzing a problem to find its solution is like trying to restore freshness to a leaf by treating the leaf itself, whereas the solution lies in watering the root."*

So, let's focus on the root of who you really are which is pure wellness and aligned with your soul's purpose. That is definitely the top floor for our elevator. Let's focus in this positive upward direction. So, let me share with you this revolutionary tool and then let's have some fun with it.

Visualize the *BGOOD4U Awakening Map* as if it were a building. You enter the building at the intersection point of the "+" at the horizontal *Neutral* line. From this ground floor you have easy open access to the mezzanine which is the *Satisfaction* floor. You can either take the stairs or the elevator up to the right, but you can see this second floor (the first floor above the neutral lobby) from the entrance. It is almost as if it is one big two-story floor.

From the lobby you can go to the left and access the elevator to the basement floors. When you get in the F (Fear) Elevator the first floor below ground level is *Courage*. From that elevator you have access to the following floors in descending order: *Pessimism, Frustration, Overwhelm, Disappointment, Doubt, Worry, Blame, Anger, Revenge, Jealousy, Unworthiness, Fear, Grief, Apathy, Depression, Guilt* and ending with *Shame* at the very bottom floor.

Now from the lobby you can also go to the right and access the elevator to the top floors. When you get in the L (Love) Elevator the first floor above ground level is *Satisfaction* that you can also reach via the open stairway in the lobby. Then from the L Elevator, the floor above *Satisfaction* is *Willingness* and from there in the L elevator

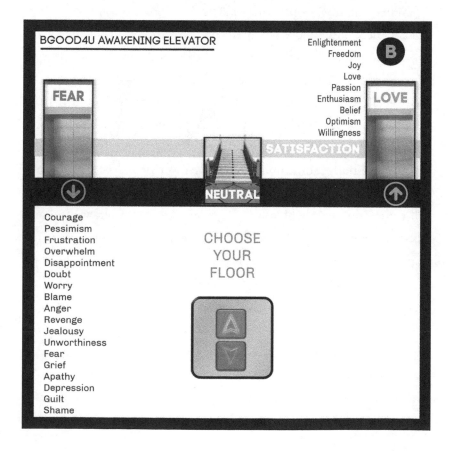

you have access to the following floors in ascending order: *Optimism, Belief, Enthusiasm, Passion, Love, Joy, Freedom, and Enlightenment* at the very top floor. You could also put Bliss at the top floor with your point B along with your soul's purpose.

You can't reach any of the top floors from the F elevator. The highest you can reach for is *Neutral* and *Satisfaction* from the F elevator. The only way to get to those top floors is take the baby steps up past all the lower floors to at least *Neutral* or *Satisfaction*. From there you can walk over to the L elevator to get to the higher floors of where you want to go.

When the doors open on a particular floor, you get to peek at what is there and choose whether you want to get off on that floor. You get to choose whether you want to spend more time there or whether you want to go to a better feeling higher floor. Each floor above feels better than the one below even in the F elevator. Each floor above is more powerful than the one below too with the most powerful being the *Enlightenment* floor.

You will notice some floors may have more people that you know, or they may be familiar because it is where you used to live but you still get to choose on which floor you want to stop, walk around and talk to people. It is only up to you. People may be calling your name from that floor or wanting to show you something or you may see something horrific that gets your attention but still it is just you that gets to choose on which floor you actually want to spend more time.

What you will notice is that if you are on the *Apathy/Depression* floors and you decide you've had enough of that and you manage to make your way to the elevator doors, past everyone else who wants you to stay on their floor, and you actually press the up elevator button, you already feel a little better. And if you stop off on the

Anger floor for a little bit you will notice that this feels even better. Because if you have been feeling powerless and apathetic, it feels a little bit great, to get a little bit mad and get your power back. Although you don't want to stay stuck here when there are so many more great levels to reach. Now if you were on the *Love* floor and are now on the *Anger* floor, that feels worse. It feels worse to go down and it feels worse to lose your power and it feels worse to go in the opposite direction of your soul's purpose.

So, when we look at the elevators, it is crystal clear that we can't get to what we want through guilt, unworthiness, jealousy, anger, blame or even overwhelm and frustration. This is something that took me decades to realize. We can run around and work like crazy on the anger or frustration floor and literally get nowhere. And sometimes, someone can get on our elevator and push the button to a really low floor that they are choosing (without even knowing it) and it can be tempting to go there with them, but you don't have to do that.

Now there are some bonuses to this elevator, and you can get a key card—an express pass that takes you right up to *Neutral* and *Satisfaction* without stopping on every floor if you are in the F elevator and brings you up to all of the penthouse suite floors on the L elevator. You can get these express passes with meditation and sleep and a few other ways that we will go into in more detail in Chapter 9.

Alright, so this may seem like a cute clever little metaphor, but how can we actually use it? Well if I am on my computer and it stops working—maybe I get the whirling color ball of doom on my Mac or maybe I can't open something because I forgot the most recent change of password and let's say I feel myself slipping into frustration. If I decide to choose to feel frustrated by this, sure enough more comes my way to feel frustrated about, and I realize—ugh! I got off on the Frustration floor. Now I can continue and then even notice that there are some people that I must get back to that I haven't yet. And then my kids will ask me for clothes that I haven't washed yet. And then my credit card on some monthly important expense is expired. And then the dog starts barking. And then I will notice a talk I am supposed to be giving that I haven't started on yet and then I realize— ugh! I got off on the Overwhelm floor. Now sometimes I will try and work harder in the Frustration and Overwhelm floors thinking that this will help me get out but—decades of experience with this futile approach, I now know better! And I know that this now aptly named "F" elevator can be a slippery slope into the basement that starts to ripple out and impact the world around me and the ones I love. And I can really feel "F'd."

So, what can I do when I feel like I am going in the wrong direction and accidentally take the F elevator instead of the L? Well noticing that you are in the wrong elevator is a great first step. That is huge! The majority of the population doesn't know this yet. They don't know they have a choice and that it does matter. So, remember the most we have access to is Neutral and Satisfaction from the F elevator. We aren't capable of feeling ecstatic from there. So, you want to focus on something that will bring you to the Neutral or Satisfaction floors.

When I got the news that my dad had his stroke, I focused on laundry—a very neutral subject. When I had just finished scanning a newborn baby that had died, I focused on the cool water that was washing my hands afterward, that was neutral with a twinge of satisfaction. Most people don't. They focus on the problem and what isn't working without realizing that actually makes the problem worse and gives them more of the same on that floor that they are inadvertently choosing. The lower floors are extremely crowded. But as my parents taught me that just because everyone else is doing it, that doesn't make it right. As I mentioned previously, I get that this is a lot easier said than done when you are counteracting a lifetime of lower floor living and when everyone else is doing it, but it doesn't have to be that way and if you really want to help someone, you will choose to elevate yourself to the higher floors where all of your power is.

I noticed in my early days, health coaching that the better I was, the better my clients were. If I was going through a rough patch so were they. This is when I first came up with my saying "Be Good For You" because the better I was, the better they were and then selfishly as I taught them this, the better they were, the better I was.

Recently I found myself slipping into the Frustration floor with my computer stalling and some house renovations that were not done that I was focusing on (instead of what was working). Then I received an email from a doctor interested in my program (which should be a great thing) but he wasn't really my ideal client. He had tons of questions in his email and I could tell he was frustrated and skeptical. I gave him a link to my calendar to discuss because then I could answer what his *real* questions were. But still as he sent more emails with more questions before we even had our appointment, I was starting to feel frustrated and began to regret inviting him to speak with me, when I would really prefer to focus on writing this book and helping those who want to be helped. I could see how I had rendezvoused with him on the Frustration floor that I let my computer issues take me to. So now what? I could continue on the Frustration floor and answer his many time-consuming questions (which he didn't know yet but were really the wrong questions) or I could change my state. I decided on the latter. I was tired so I took a thirty-minute nap. Then when I got up, I meditated for fifteen minutes. Then I loved on my dog (that almost always works) and then I focused on serving my clients who I absolutely love! After I was done serving my clients, I noticed that I had another email. The doctor who had booked the appointment just cancelled. Problem solved without me doing anything. Perfect! I literally no longer had access to him on the Frustration floor now that I was in the Love elevator.

We can't change certain circumstances and many of us have had and will have some major ones, but we can change what we focus on and we can choose to focus onward and upward at least to get to *Neutral* as I did with my dad initially with focusing on the laundry. Then *Willingness* as I read that book about the brain's way of healing. Then *Optimism* as my dad was off oxygen and we had some little wins of the day for post-it notes. Then *Belief* as he started to stand. Until ultimately, we had a full-on miracle in the making as I stood firmly in the upper floors of the *Love* elevator, refusing to get on the F elevator. Not now. The stakes were way too high. I didn't dare.

So, what about when the stakes aren't high? It is way easier to catch yourself early in the elevator to the Frustration floor before you step foot onto that floor. So, we have talked about meditation and we are going to talk about that some more in upcoming chapters but what is a simple thing that you can do right now to move you up the elevator?

As I shared in the previous examples, choosing to focus on something neutral or satisfying is huge, and it does not have to be on the same subject and often you can't find something satisfying on the same subject. So, I can't find anything satisfying about being told that my dad has suffered a massive stroke and will not live, and I am miles away not knowing if I can get there on time. But I can focus on laundry—which may to you seem so disrespectful—but I know it was this and thousands of other little decisions like that—that led to my dad's miraculous recovery. Most of the world is not ready to hear this yet. I know that. They are in the bottom floors and can't imagine that life could ever be wonderful and if it is, that is for other people who "lucked out." That is not how it is at all. But I appreciate if this is a major paradigm shift and that if you look out across the horizon and see evidence that the world is flat that you can't possibly believe that the world is round. And as you look out over the floor you are on which is not what you want—which may not have enough money or health or love or happiness—it may seem impossible that you have a choice. But you do! This is why I am so excited about sharing this with you! This is my life's work! This is what I am really meant to do! To connect people like you with what they really want—to their soul's purpose—and show you how to "Be Good For You"!

So some satisfying things that I think about to uplift me when I stumble onto Frustration (this is not about being perfect) is the sunshine, the comfort of my pillow, my favorite coffee mug, the trees gently blowing outside in the breeze, drinking water, my dog, the feel of water on my skin, walking through the woods, the softness of my hair, the warmth of my home. Anything that you feel satisfied about works. From Chapter 3, you made a list of times when you felt most alive and what you love to do. Refer to that list and see if there is any quick go to activity that you can do to uplift you. It may be going for a jog or taking a nap or meditating. Sometimes it is just a thirty-second pause to notice the sunshine or some favorite socks.

Literally something this simple can start to do it. But you want to keep that consistent positive focus in the right direction. So, what are some things you can put on your "go-to" list that will allow you to switch elevators?

One of my favorite ways to be proactive with the elevator and access the express pass to Satisfaction is through gratitude and appreciation. I take a journal style calendar that is a "week at a glance" and on the ten spaces for each day, write out what I am grateful for (or as I phrase it—what I appreciate). This simple daily exercise helps to keep me focused on what I do want and what is working and keeps me in the L elevator. Plus given that it is a calendar I can easily see if I missed a day and it keeps me accountable. *But* if I do miss a day or week, I do not beat myself up about it as that would place me in the F elevator getting out on the Guilt or Overwhelm floor and no good can come from that. But when you do this, watch for amazing things to happen! I remember a number of years ago, I was in a tight bubble of positivity for one week. I refused to let anyone else get on my elevator and push my buttons. I focused upward. For the three months prior, I had been writing a daily list of twenty things (instead of my usual ten) that I was grateful for. I said a mantra "Go Powerful" that I had heard that an Olympic Gold speed skater would say to herself during her race and in that positive one-week bubble, events conspired on my behalf and my income doubled in one week resulting in a six-figure annual income that year as a holistic entrepreneur (separate from my medical career). You may laugh at these little practices that have saved my dad's life and created a successful thriving life for me as a holistic entrepreneur—and I get it. There was a time this would have seemed hokey for me too. But I really want you to have amazing success and if I hold back on the secret sauce and you are left scratching your head why things aren't working for you and you don't do the amazing healing work you were meant to do—no one wins. Plus, I know that if anyone is ready and able to hear this it is holistic entrepreneurs. Test it out for yourself. Just beware of judging too soon like I shared in Chapter 5 and remember if you are frustrated, disappointed, worried or doubtful—you are in the wrong elevator and no good can come from that.

This can be a really helpful tool. As I coach one of my clients that works in a very busy hospital, where she has a lot of negative interactions with co-workers, before she engages, she now thinks about what floor she is choosing. We have a few strategies to choose an alternate floor like going to the washroom and focusing on the water. Staring at the computer screen and doing some silent breathing and thinking of her "go to" list are a few of her other strategies that are working extremely well and as Wayne Dyer said, "When you change the way you look at things, the things you look at change."

As you start to create your world-class signature program, keep this *BGOOD4U Awakening Elevator* in mind. There will be plenty of opportunity to come from love or fear. Choose love. There will be plenty of opportunity to stay stuck on floors where you have spent the most time but choose to elevate yourself as best you can. Begin to incorporate daily little practices like appreciation lists, wins of the day and make a "go to" list right now of some things you can do or think about to move you up in the elevator. In the next chapter, now that you are coming from an elevated place of love, you are going to build out the specifics of your world-class signature program!

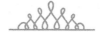

Chapter 8

Name the Steps in Your Signature Program

"The vision must be followed by the venture. It is not enough to stare up the steps—we must step up the stairs."
–Vance Havner

This next step is really exciting because your signature program is now taking shape and coming to life! Grab a pen and your notebook, and here we go! Write down your ideal client's specific problem at the top of your page. Then at the bottom of the page, write down the specific result *they* want in *their* words. This is their dream come true or at least the part of their dream come true that you can deliver. Just above their solution, write what you want them to get out of your program—what they *really* need that they may not even know that they need yet.

For example, your client may have a problem with asthma and their dream come true may be to breathe easy so they don't have to worry if they forgot their inhaler on a date. Now you may want them to know that there are certain foods that are triggering their asthma, but they don't even know that foods have anything to do with that yet. So, breathing easy and being symptom-free is the result they want. Teaching them what foods trigger their asthma is what you want them to know. You will both get what you want but it is important to know this distinction because you are going to be attracting them and speaking to them in language they can hear, so they can find you in the jungle. You still get to deliver the "real" solution to them. However, if you start with that (allergenic foods, self-love, etc.) you won't attract them because they don't even know they need to know that yet.

Knowing what problem your clients are looking for is critical. One of my clients Jennifer, who had experienced and journeyed through her own premature birth of her son, really wanted to help women prevent premature births. But no one was looking for that because obviously, you don't know it is going to happen to you until it does and then it is too late. I could relate to that. I started out wanting to prevent cancer (and honestly, not just any cancer—but my grandmother's cancer which wasn't possible). But no one actually cared because they didn't think it would happen to them. I could talk about clean eating, but they didn't see this as a problem they needed to solve, especially ten to fifteen years ago before people really started to awaken to the role that their food choices had upon their cancer risk. Plus, as a healer wanting to prevent cancer, how would I know if I was successful? If no one got cancer, how would I know I made a difference? How would we know if they were actually going to get a cancer or not?

Instead, I looked at what problem my ideal clients were looking to solve—and that was weight loss! That was something they were actively looking for and investing time, money, and attention to solve. That is one of the reasons my focus was weight loss for more than fifteen years. I had solved this for myself. I could help them solve it and, in the process, I could deliver great anti-inflammatory foods and practices infused with self-love so that—maybe, just maybe—I could have a role in preventing cancer. We will never know.

So, to solve this for Jennifer, we focused on her areas of expertise and why she was passionate about this and what she could help women with that they were already actively looking to solve. Through our discussion, we realized that polycystic ovarian syndrome was something that she had studied extensively and was a doorway through which she could help these women. They were actively looking for a solution as to what they could do to counteract the increased risk of infertility, weight gain, facial hair, and (what they often didn't know they were also at risk for...) premature births! Jennifer now had a specific niche that she could serve that was actively looking for information she could provide, and in the meantime, she still got to deliver what she really wanted (that satisfied her soul)—to prevent premature births! You still can serve with your message that you were meant to share, but we need to language it in a way that your ideal clients can hear, otherwise neither of you can find each other hiding in the jungle.

A common thing that most healers want to "solve" is to teach people to love themselves. Granted, that is actually the route to heal as evidenced by the Love elevator and map, but you only know that *after* you have solved your problem. My client Nicole came to me and said that teaching self-love was what she really felt called to do and she had lots of compelling reasons why this was important to her. However, I reminded her that people who don't love themselves (most people) aren't looking to hire someone to help them with that because ... they don't think they are lovable! So, you are then left with no clients and may even start to doubt your own self-worth. As we went through a process like I just outlined with Jennifer, we realized that she was able to help someone keep off nearly 100 pounds for five years post bariatric surgery! She didn't think that was a big deal because she felt like the surgery played the role in weight loss, when in fact Nicole was a certified holistic health coach with extensive nutritional knowledge and it is very clear that without changing overall lifestyle habits and mindset, the weight would almost certainly have been regained. But Nicole also knew the critical role self-love played in results as she observed many people's lives which led to her strong desire to teach this (to satisfy her soul).

Once again, her "behind the ear niche" that was so close to her she couldn't recognize it, was also a perfect fit to satisfy her soul. Patients who undergo bariatric surgery (and those who don't) often lack in the self-love department. There is at some level a lack of belief that they can lose the weight "on their own" in time and there is a need for Nicole's skills. Because without the nutritional and mindset upgrade, the statistics support regaining the weight. These patients are actively looking to keep the weight off with their new lease on life and may even have some feelings of guilt or shame (which we already know won't get them to their happily ever after). So, with this refined specific niche of supporting bariatric surgery patients to long term weight loss/maintenance which is what they are looking for, Nicole still can deliver what is in her healer's heart to teach—self-love!

Once you are now crystal clear on your parameters: your ideal client, their problem, their dream come true and what you want them to receive, write down the steps that your client must go through or the things they need to know to be able to go from point A (their current problem) to point B (their dream come true). What is the absolute best way that you know of at this point to get your clients from point A to point B? Always keep delivering your best. You will continue to learn and evolve but bring your best that you can right now. Ask yourself what the critical information is your clients must have to get from point A to point B. This isn't about adding fluff. It is about giving them all of the puzzle pieces they require with no extra pieces and no missing pieces. What is the logical process you are walking them through? Then divide this journey into five to ten categories or steps or modules (no fewer than three and no more than twelve). The number of steps should closely align with the weeks in your program (with perhaps an additional orientation or celebration week).

The way I like to do this is via a process I call a "post-it brain dump." It is how I used to study in university, medical school and residency. It is how I created websites and it is what I teach to my health professional clients. When faced with a large overwhelming mountain of information, I learned to categorize it all into broad categories and then divide and conquer each category and then focus and finish each particular step of that category. It is amazing how much information you can manage when it is organized and how it brings clarity to the entire process. I like to use big blank sheets of paper that are the back of old desk calendars (20" x 14") and colored post-it notes. I pick the broad categories and assign a particular color. For example, your categories may be: Mindset (yellow), Nutrition (orange), Activity (pink), Theory (blue), Action Steps (green), Case Studies (red). Then I will write the steps or items they need to know or do to get their results on the appropriate colored post-it. How you organize your program will vary depending on your niche and format. For example, an online course may have the categories as above or maybe each week when you are coaching someone you start with a step that includes the required mindset, nutrition, activity, theory and action step and supporting case study for them to take their next step. Then the following week it follows the same format but takes it to the next deeper level *or* perhaps it just covers another food, mindset, activity, etc.

Displaying your post-it notes on the big sheet allows a great overview visual and allows you to easily play around with the items you want to teach to determine the best order to teach them. You can use other ways to organize your information depending on how tech savvy you are. A few that I also regularly use are Trello, Evernote, and Workflowy. Check them out if you are so inclined. These options do have the benefit of being able to copy and paste your work over into actual online course modules. However, honestly, I still almost always start out with my big old calendars (I buy last year's in December or January just for this reason or large blank sheets). I also like large giant whiteboards to organize information too. But still for me, nothing like being able to move around a colored post-it. Trello would be the closest digital equivalent to post-its if you like things techier.

In determining your categories, this is where you will call upon your experience in problem solving your ideal client's problem. How did you solve it for yourself or your clients? What is the best way that you know for your clients to get the very best result? In addition, as you invite clients to your beta program and are coaching them while you are creating this program, your clients will help you make it better. For example, as my client Tim started coaching and training his clients he recommended as one of the early steps, green smoothies and some other nutritional tips. This led his clients to ask for green smoothie recipes. So now within his program, these recipes are a resource that he will be including. Sometimes we think our clients know what we know, and we forget how far we've come ourselves. This is why I recommend coaches start coaching one-on-one initially because you will learn so much about what the missing links are, what questions they have and what resonates most with them. Eventually however as we talked about previously, depending on your income goals, you likely will want to find a way to offset trading time for money. This is what transforms your practice from a straight health coaching practice with forty-five- to sixty-minute sessions with no set curriculum to a signature program. A health coaching practice with no set curriculum can definitely work to achieve results but there is a ceiling on your income eventually because there is a finite amount of your time in a day. This may or may not be an issue. This model has the lowest initial start-up costs. You don't necessarily even need a website or any physical or online overhead costs and is a great place to start—even perhaps the first baby step with your initial beta clients as you create your signature program. However, if you are the sole income earner looking to leave or replace a medical career income, this is not likely to be enough.

I love to supplement the value I can deliver to my clients with an online course or curriculum. This can take many forms. It can be like my Meal Cure membership site where I create five quick and easy thirty-minute healthy dinner recipes each week with a weekly organized grocery list and superfood video on the food of the week. This is information that I create once and then can be delivered to multiple people at a time and they can access at their own convenience. This was in response to a question I frequently was asked by my clients (and myself): "What's for dinner?" This was a way to deliver additional relevant helpful information to my clients and leverage myself.

Other typical online courses can be structured into modules where clients can get the baseline information and then to increase connection and accountability, additionally offer a weekly group (or individual) Q&A call. This is my favorite way of serving clients and how I design my signature programs. It is the best of both worlds. They receive a lot of "me" in the online videos and slides without it taking up all of my time. They can access the modules at their convenience and replay and pause as much as they want. Then they have a basic understanding and we work closely on our weekly video calls (currently I use Zoom) to implement what is taught in the modules and answer questions and coach through any mindset blocks.

You can use this latter format to create your initial beta program that eventually becomes your signature program. As you teach your content at the beginning of the zoom call, this can be recorded for future use when you run your program again or even as a bonus once you are at a new level with your program. After the teaching portion, you can open the call to discussion and questions (even off of recording) which is the best part. The reason I like the first iteration of your program done this way is because your clients are all at the same stage together and they can learn from each other. Your future version of your signature program however will benefit from your original beta clients' questions and input. You can still structure your signature program, so your clients are all at the same point in the process if that makes sense. Alternatively, you can have a rolling enrolment as in a weight loss program where people can just start anytime when they are ready, and it is fine that they are at different stages in the group.

Once you have your five to ten steps in your program, I recommend creating video lessons for each step. This is not mandatory, but it is a great way to convey information. Even if you choose to continue a solely one-to-one practice, I recommend creating power point slides or private video lessons even if it is just for you with your phone. This forces you to get clear on your messaging and helps to define your curriculum and steps that are required to bring your client from point A to B rather than just meeting each week to "hang out." Having said that, do not underestimate the value of time spent in silence with your client. Their biggest "aha" moments and breakthroughs are the ones they come to realize on their own. But you can lead them right up to that point so they can see it for themselves. This is again why I like the didactic teaching component to be online, so that when I am with my client in session, I can spend more time listening to them and actually coaching, knowing that they have all the resources they require in the online component of the signature program. There is also a greater perceived (and real) value when you offer a "tangible" course *plus* you—the expert.

So, go ahead and outline the logical steps of your program. You can name them with a pneumonic like I have done with the *Awakening Process* but it is not necessary. Sometimes that makes it awkward. Only do this if it still works in the best interest of your client. But regardless name your steps and name your signature program! You may already know the name you want for your program, but it should reflect what you do. We will talk more about naming your program in Chapter 11, but it may be clear to you at this point what your program wants to be called. But for this chapter definitely outline and name your steps. I recommend naming them according to the topic of the week or module. It could be greens week or beans week or self-care week, etc. This will be the topic of teaching that week although of course people will be eating greens, beans, and doing self-care each week but this allows a nice organized framework for your program. Structure brings a welcome clarity to your client where they can see their progression through your program to their desired destination. Each of the steps are the factors that will influence their success. In the next chapter, as you begin to launch and implement your signature program, we are going to identify *your* influencers that influence *your* success!

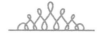

Chapter 9

Identify Your Influencers

"You are the master of your destiny. You can influence, direct and control your own environment. You can make your life what you want it to be."

–Napoleon Hill

A s we begin to fill in the details of your signature program so that you can maximize the success of your ideal clients, it is the perfect time to pull back the curtains on the details that maximize *your own* success. Have you ever wondered why two people can have very similar credentials on paper and one is massively successful and the other never actually launches? We are going to delve into the idea of what I call your magnetic influencers that are another key ingredient in the secret sauce!

Recall from Chapter 3, the introduction to the *BGOOD4U Awakening Map* which was the precursor to the elevator. I want you to imagine that "+" on the map with your positive destination in the top right corner and guilt, shame, doubt, and frustration in the negative left lower quadrant. As we consider these various emotional states, I also want you to recall times in your life when you were really on a roll. Things were just clicking and there was an element of ease to it—even if just briefly and you were getting right up there with enthusiasm, passion, love, and joy. There was an element of momentum that was carrying you. Now I am sure you can also recall times when everything was hitting the fan and you were in a tailspin in the negative direction and there just wasn't much you could do as things just went from bad to worse. Again, there was an element of momentum at play.

At the extreme ends of the map, whether you are in an upward spiral or downward spiral there is momentum, and life tends to conspire on your behalf (or against you). So as things get better for you in this journey to create your signature program (or lose weight or make a living or overcome dis-ease), it may be slow at the beginning with the baby steps but then, provided that you keep focused in the positive direction, they will get easier and easier, better and better. On the other hand, as you go in the negative direction, it is way better to nip it in the bud right away when you first notice you are in frustration or overwhelm or doubt rather than dwelling in the lower floors because you can swiftly find yourself in some really dark places that take a lot more effort and focus to overcome. I speak from personal experience and I am very certain you have had times in your life when you can attest to this yourself. So that is why I am very careful to notice where I am on the map and what floor I am choosing and coach my clients to notice the same. That is why when old patterns of fear or frustration are triggered, I do what I can to choose a better feeling thought or area of focus. Often the best you can do is neutral or at most satisfaction as I have shared before with noticing sunshine or your pillow or that your heart is still beating.

But there are also magnetic influencers that can influence your position on the map too. Certainly, you will have noticed that there are certain circumstances in which it is easier than others to be more positive and that are more conducive to your success. I want you to imagine a large magnet at the top right corner of the map pulling you onward and upward as well as a large magnet at the bottom left corner of the map dragging you down. There are seven broad categories of magnetic influencers:

1. People
2. Environment
3. Activity
4. Food
5. Thoughts
6. Beliefs
7. Choices

Some people that surround you are conducive to your success and extremely supportive while others are toxic and sabotaging. This actually has a huge influence upon you and likely more than you appreciate. *As the iconic motivational speaker Jim Rohn once said, "You are the average of the five people you spend the most time with."*

The five people you spend the most time with often have similar incomes, eating habits, weight, and opinions. The fastest way to improve your results is to hang around with people who have the results you want (rather than those that are complaining about their results they don't want). It is also important to remember that there will be definitely times when the only person who believes in you is—you. So, you don't want to be dependent on these people, but it can be helpful to surround yourself more of the time with people who are a positive influence rather than a negative.

The same can be said for your environment. A noisy or chaotic or war-torn environment is going to have a different effect upon you than a quiet, clear or peaceful environment. Different activities that you do also can positively or negatively influence you—including sleep, meditation, exercise and various habits.

A large portion of my coaching has focused on the influence of food upon our mood and behavior and success. Certainly, we have all observed the obvious effect of excess alcohol, caffeine or sugar upon someone's behavior and mood. But even tiny details as to where or how or by whom the food was prepared can have a different effect upon every aspect of us. Consider organic versus artificial. Consider someone who is a cattle rancher versus a vegan. You can imagine that their diet influences the way they look and feel. If you have ever changed your diet significantly and noticed that you felt differently— more or less mental clarity—more or less energy—more or less headaches or body discomfort, then you have observed the incredible power of food because after all we truly are what we eat. Every one of our hundred trillion cells is made up of the building blocks we feed it. We are DNA wrapped in food. So, it is no surprise that as these building blocks form our cells and hormones, that they are going to influence how we think and feel. So, we all know the obvious extremes of how we think when we have a lot of alcohol or caffeine.

But even at the subtlest levels, food (although often not appreciated) actually influences our thoughts. And our thoughts do matter. There is definitely a difference between positive and encouraging optimistic thoughts and fearful, negative, guilty, doubting, self-sabotaging thoughts upon the direction that we are moving in life.

There are other factors, apart from food, that determine our thoughts. Certainly, most thoughts run repeat patterns based on our experience and observations and form our beliefs. These beliefs are greatly determined in our early years by those around us although they can be changed. If it was expected that we would succeed or that we would fail, most often we comply with these beliefs as our default setting.

Finally, and most importantly is the influence of choices that we make upon the direction that we move on our map. Of course, there is choice in all of the above factors, but there is also a choice in terms of where we direct our attention. For example, we can choose to watch negative news or comedies. We can choose to learn something new or choose to consider a different perspective or not.

Here are some common powerful positive influencers that act like a magnet pulling you up to your desired outcome that you may want to increase:

- Meditation
- Deep Breathing
- Drinking water
- Sleep
- Nutrition that nourishes you
- Activity you enjoy
- Conditions* that please you

Here are some common powerful negative influencers that act like a magnet dragging you down away from your desired outcome:

- Negative news, ads, articles, and posts
- Discouraging diagnosis
- Dehydration
- Sleep deprivation
- Lack of nourishment
- Stress
- Conditions* that displease you

You will notice an * by the word "conditions." This is because all of us can be influenced to feel better or worse under certain conditions. However, you *always have a choice* as to how you choose to feel under any circumstance. *Always!* If you need the conditions to be different for you to feel good, you are in trouble. In other words, if we are in the F elevator in these bottom dweller floors and we need the floors to change for us to get to the Love elevator…that never happens! Life does not work that way. Expecting someone else to redecorate the Frustration floor for us so it is not frustrating won't happen. Wanting someone else to press the "button" to the Satisfaction or Joy "floors" won't happen. The bad news is we get to choose for ourselves. I am not saying it is easy to choose the positive thought at all. When I was told that my dad could not survive, it would have been easier to choose the default pattern of most which is fear and grief or even guilt for moving away from parents as they were getting older. Let's say you launch a program, and no one shows up right away for your event or offer and maybe there was a glitch that happened that you want to blame for the failure. It is easier to choose the default of blame or that what you are doing isn't working or that you don't know enough or that this will never work. But if you choose to focus positively and find something (and it doesn't have to be about your program and maybe it can't be some days) to find some measure of satisfaction to get you pointed in the L elevator, this will make all the difference in the world.

When my dad was first taken by ambulance with his massive stroke, my mom was in the ambulance with him. No one said anything. She was whisked into a hospital family room alone as soon as they took my dad into emergency. She sat there for hours with no word. She got a phone call while she was there from the very hospital she was at, indicating that my dad had been taken to hospital (which of course she knew) and that they had his dentures. My mom said that she was at that hospital in the family room. They said okay. They came and gave her my dad's dentures and left. That was it. She didn't know if there was more of him to come. Was that all that was left of him? Much later the doctor came and told her that he was sorry, but my dad's stroke was far too massive and there was nothing they could (past tense "could" screamed out at her) do for him. They then said that they had already transferred him to the community hospital (of course leaving my mom with no ride home too). They said he was not conscious, would not recognize us, and he could not survive.

So, under these horrible *conditions*, what did my mom *choose* to do? Instead of anger or worry or blame, she *chose* to focus on appreciation and gratitude as she wrote out a list of things that she was grateful for—that my dad was not in pain and that he had a great life and that we have a great family. She wasn't doing this to coerce conditions or to get a different result. She didn't know a different result was possible. The doctors had told her there was not. But from a place of love for her grandchildren and in trying to explain what was happening to her grandchildren, she gathered her thoughts from a place of positive focus and firmly laid the foundation for the medical miracle that was about to unfold.

The successful launching of a signature program is a heck of a lot easier than orchestrating a medical miracle and defying all the odds—that is of course, if you have a strong, positive desire in the forward direction regardless of conditions—regardless of your current circumstances. Think of how many celebrities and success stories you have heard who started from nothing. Everyone starts somewhere. People and conditions are going to try to discourage and distract you. Guard your focus like it is a suitcase with a million dollars. You can always create another million dollars with your forward focus but without forward focus you are left to the whims of everyone else if you let everyone and everything have power and influence over you. Don't let others rent space in your head. Don't psyche yourself out if you are starting at zero or facing seemingly unsurmountable odds. And we all have moments where we feel like this—where we feel like our back is up against the wall and there is no way out. That is okay. That is normal. Don't beat yourself up and go to the blame, guilt, shame side of the map. But catch yourself early and notice what floor you are choosing before momentum takes over and you are in a huge tailspin that makes it a lot harder (although not impossible) to recover.

Alright so we know we are in control of how we choose to feel (even if this concept is new for you, it will be a lot more empowering as you test it out than assuming someone else has control over you and you are helpless—which is not true). But there are influencers we can choose to make this journey a lot easier to succeed. The five most common influencers that have impacted my life and my clients' lives are the following:

1. Meditation
2. Stress
3. Sleep
4. Superfoods
5. Water

Each of these I talk about in more detail in my BGOOD4U Facebook group and in my YouTube videos and with my clients, but here is a quick summary. Meditation we have discussed previously but the reason why this is so powerful is that it allows you to hook up with what you really want and who you really are. There is a natural tendency for things to work out for us and move us in the positive direction. Our bodies thrive despite ourselves (I was always amazed as a medical student about this). If we just stop focusing in the opposite direction, we will naturally at least get to neutral. Meditation and quieting the mind allow us to stop the often-incessant negative chatter in our heads even just briefly. This has the effect of a magnet pulling you up to your destination. Meditating for fifteen minutes once or twice a day can be life-changing but often this is noticed more retrospectively. Often there isn't some massive change in fifteen minutes. It usually feels like nothing at all. But if you look back over a few months or years, you will absolutely be amazed as to how things worked out. My clients are often amazed as their clients coincidentally "show up" in their experience in the most wonderful ways that they could not have predicted or how opportunities opened up for them.

Stress is our number one killer. It is at the root of all dis-ease. It increases our cortisol, our blood sugars, our blood pressure, our inflammation, our belly fat, our heart disease, and cancer, and autoimmune disease, etc. We can't always do anything to change the stressor in the moment, but we can do things like meditation and nutrition to allow our bodies to respond better. For instance, adaptogen herbs are substances that help our bodies physically adapt to stress. These are things like ashwagandha and shilajit. I go into more details about the foods to consider and avoid in my groups but certainly nutrition plays a major role. Minimizing the stressful situation always helps. Choosing a different floor helps. Most people fan the flames of stress and inflame it further. Something awful happens and then they post all about it over and over, and they tell the story of their injustice to their friends over and over and stay right on the floor where that occurred opening themselves up to more of the same. Or sometimes it is a private stress. Maybe it is body shaming or overwhelming debt or a horrible illness or grief that has them gripped firmly in the clutches of stress. Again, do your best to baby step yourself up that tiny bit. Inch yourself forward that little bit. Find something else to focus upon.

I once heard a medical doctor on TV state that she cured herself of her breast cancer by watching comedies almost nightly and watching no news at all, improving her nutrition with many greens and being in bed by 10:00 p.m. These simple things may seem silly, but they are really powerful. Many people *choose* to work themselves into a knot over a relationship or political situation or some other stressor and no good can ever come of that. You can't get mad enough to help people be happy. You can't get scared enough to feel at ease. You can't get sick enough to help people be well. You can't get poor enough to help people be wealthy. Your only hope in improving the situation I have discovered from my personal experience and coaching thousands of others is to "be good for you."

Sleep is obviously an important part of our wellness and like meditation, if nothing else, it allows us to take a reprieve from beating up on ourselves. In all transparency, this is the one that I am the least great at. Years studying and pulling all-nighters, sleepless nights on call, sleepless nights as a mom of four sons in less than six years and then trying to develop as a holistic entrepreneur while working as a physician was a perfect set up for this. I truly believe I can get away with less sleep than most people. I am not sure which came first—whether this was innate or developed out of decades of necessity to function. However, I love sleeping and I do it a lot more now, although I still can get right into a passion project and completely enjoy working away into the wee hours. This does not at all feel like previous tossing and turning nights trying to "figure things out." There is a difference. However, we all do need sleep. It is great for our health and it is great for our business. It allows for mental clarity. When we "let it go" while we sleep, we often become inspired to great ideas. I will get some of my best insights as I am falling asleep or waking up. If you are well rested, you will be a better coach. If you are exhausted your clients will not be getting your best. You cannot fill from an empty cup. Sleep will be important to address with your clients too as it is a big determinant to health.

I have written on superfoods extensively including my book *Doctor Up the Recipe* and have recorded many YouTube videos on superfoods on my *Dr Shaunna* channel. Choose foods that help you be good for you. Notice how you feel when you eat certain foods. If you are at optimal health and mental clarity, your signature program and business will thrive too.

Finally, the simplest thing to incorporate for most people is water. This is often where I start with my private coaching clients. Just drinking water is hugely impactful for weight loss, improved circulation, better skin, mental clarity and youthful energy. In creating your signature programs, remembering to stay well hydrated is important in creating the mental clarity and energy to create your program and attract and sustain your clients.

As you become one of the five people that your clients will spend the most time with in your program, you have an opportunity to be a great positive influencer acting as a magnet to lift your clients up to the best version of themselves as you lift yourself up. Be aware of the factors that positively influence you and also some of the negative influencers where you may want to choose to direct less attention.

Write down a list of your "go to" positive influencers that can lift you up:

1. Who are the people?
2. Where are the places?
3. What are the activities?
4. What are your nourishing foods?
5. What are the positive thoughts?
6. What are the supportive beliefs?
7. What choices do you want to *choose* to positively influence your success and counteract any negative drag?

In the next chapter, you are going to want to have this list handy and regularly incorporate these items as we look at the best ways to nurture your clients and yourself. Ramping up your positive influencers and diminishing your negative influencers will allow you to more easily direct your focus so that you have the right mindset to hold the space for amazing transformations for your clients and of course, for you to allow yourself to receive the natural success spinoffs—physically, financially, and emotionally.

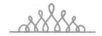

Chapter 10

Nurture Your Clients and Yourself

"Wealth, like happiness, is never attained when sought after directly. It comes as a by-product of providing a useful service."
–Henry Ford

The absolute beauty of a truly soul-satisfying signature program the way that we have been creating it is that it definitely nourishes you—because you have designed it to be in alignment with what you really want, serving the people you want to serve, solving the problems you want to solve and it is truly an extension of who you are. But also, because you have designed it to be in alignment with solving the specific problem that your ideal client really wants solved, it nourishes and transforms them too. It is a beautiful win-win.

It is important to have the mechanics and the mindset to launch your signature program so that it can move beyond theoretical to become an amazing vehicle that nurtures you and your client. A vehicle that allows you to make a difference and a living doing what you love. That is no small feat and hardly anyone does this. It is one thing to awaken to what you really want but it is another to be able to actually do it so that you don't have to choose between making a living and living. We have already covered many key concepts that trip people up as they try to create their programs. Your signature program already has made "better health and happiness" into something tangible that your ideal clients want and can find. I often say—it has to have "teeth" and not just be "vanilla" (I don't even know why I use this mixed metaphor, but my clients seem to get the solid versus gas nature of what I am saying here so I included it for you, too).

Okay great. Doing everything we've outlined so far; your signature program should be a sure win! But it is not. So, what is the number one thing that trips up coaches just before the finish line? Money! Ugh the "money thing." Yup. You beautiful loving healer—*you*. You generous, giving, nurturing being. What is the one thing that makes it all awkward? What is the one thing that makes your heart race and your face flush? What is the one thing that has you turn around and run into the Fear elevator? What is the underlying reason you want to hide or not put yourself out there? What is the reason you went into "health" rather than "business?" You want to heal and avoid the whole money issue. Most healers don't want to ask for money. So, we want to clean up this whole money mindset so that you can actually receive all of the abundance that you so richly desire and deserve— you beautiful, loving, professional, holistic entrepreneur—you. This way you can actually sustain the amazing healing work that you will deliver to your clients with your signature program. This way you can actually enjoy your life and your family and not have to work around the clock and put yourself and your family at risk. This really matters. We want to ensure you are choosing that win-win rather than the lose-lose alternative.

Something so beautiful as your program and the difference you will make is worth cleaning up any issues you have around money if you have them. So, what is money? It is a currency. A convenient way to lovingly exchange value. The value is set so that ideally both parties feel it is a worthy trade. You give something of value and in return they give something of value and there is a beautiful balance, and everyone feels like they are getting what they want. It is a win-win. No one *has* to buy your program and you don't *have* to let anyone inside. But when you have what they want (the specific solution to their specific problem) *and* they really, really want it solved and you are the person who can solve it, they will be willing to invest in you to help them solve it and you will find yourself on the receiving end of money. Now if they don't have that problem, don't know they have that problem, aren't looking to solve that problem, don't believe you can solve that problem or don't believe they can ever solve that problem—you may be left scratching your head wondering, where are all my ideal clients? The truth is they couldn't find you in the jungle. This is why all of the pieces we have covered so far are all little critical baby steps inching you toward this moment. So, if you are following along and you know that specific problem that your ideal clients are wanting to invest in solving, there is this one final piece that we want to make sure you have a squeaky-clean perspective—money.

The number one cause of stress overwhelmingly is finances. I've heard that an extra $500 a month could save fifty percent of marriages. I believe that is true. Money can be very triggering for people placing them in the Fear elevator and browsing the Doubt, Worry, Fear, Guilt, and Shame floors for quite some time—even a lifetime. So, you want to get the heck out of there! When you see yourself going down to those dark places—notice your floor and choose differently. Pull out your "go-to" list of influencers. Meditate. Take a nap. Focus on something you love. Focus on your clients and serving them, and less on your ego, and less on what you will look and sound like and what people are thinking of you which is none of your business. Consciously consider where you are focusing your attention. Are you focusing on what is working or what is not working? Are you focusing on where you are going or where you have been on the map? Again, I get it that this is easier said than done. But this is it. This is how it works.

Early in my coaching career, I remember giving two talks—exact same talk in two different locations within a month of each other. It was a great talk that I had put effort into delivering and marketing. I had several food props and excellent eye-opening practical content. The first talk people paid twenty-five dollars to attend. It was sold out very quickly and people received practical tips they could implement right away and some of the attendees eventually became my private clients. The other talk I gave for free...cue the crickets. Four people showed up and two of them were my parents! I still gave the talk with all of the zest I normally would to serve the people there. The following day people that had said they were going to attend the free talk but didn't, heard from the two that did attend how great it was. The non-attendees asked me when I was going to do another one.

Well—never, of course. The two people who did show up for the free talk, never did become my clients and I am not certain that talk had any lasting impact at all for them. I am embarrassed to say that I tried this experiment many times over—free coaching, free calls, etc., and it was crystal clear who got the best results—those people who actually made a commitment to invest in themselves.

You have heard it many times before and maybe you have to experience it like I did to realize people really don't value free. And they don't value cheap either. If you *really* want to make a difference and you want to allow people to commit to the program and show up consistently so they actually solve their problem and experience the magic of the transformation that your world class program delivers— you must price it accordingly so you don't unintentionally kill them with your kindness.

The financial commitment is actually part of the transformation. A clean money relationship is a loving exchange that gives your clients a way to tangibly get their results. Imagine your ideal client with their horrible problem that they really want solved. They are losing sleep over it. It is significantly negatively impacting their life. You know the solution and are willing to coach them toward their happily ever after. But if you don't offer it or they can't find your program, you can't help them. And if you don't accept their money, they don't have any place to hook their hopes and dreams onto to pull themselves up out of their problem. There is no lifeline to grab. Can you see this? Have you ever had a problem and as soon as you knew there was a solution and you decided on it and committed your time and money to it, you were already well on your way to the solution? But if they no longer offered the solution or wouldn't accept your money, how did you feel? Hopeless? Devastated? Now what were you going to do? If you don't ask for or accept your client's money, what side of the map is your client on now? Disappointed? Doubtful? Worried? What side are you on? Doubt? Unworthy? This is the lose-lose you want to avoid.

Have you ever been at a restaurant and let's say it was a special occasion you were celebrating for someone and you really wanted to pay for dinner and the other party refused? How did that feel? Rejected? Like you wanted to find another way to still pay them, like sneaking money in their jacket? On the other hand, if they let you pay for the celebration dinner and received your gift with appreciation and gratitude, how did that feel? Lovely!

When you refuse someone's gift, there is no connection or exchange that occurs. It is just two people doing their own thing. When you agree to connect and exchange value, it is a very loving act of giving and receiving. If you have trouble in the area of giving and receiving, practice it because it is definitely something that you can improve. Start by genuinely giving *and receiving* compliments every day. When you deflect the compliment with a "This old thing? That's nothing" or "No. I'm not," you reject the other person's desire to give and you reject your ability to receive and you are on the lose-lose spectrum. A simple thank you and allowing of the compliment to sink into your cells will do wonders for you and your ability to receive monetarily.

When pricing your program, of course there is the other end of the spectrum that is sometimes taught by some mentors where they tell you to just keep raising your rates without any regard for the value you are delivering, and it feels really icky and gross and the "loving exchange" feels more like a business transaction. The actual number for the optimal price for your program is going to vary depending on what value you are delivering and will almost certainly increase as you increase your experience and value in your program as you continue to deliver your best. The optimal price is somewhere above "noncommittal free" and below "grossly high repellent." That just right price is very individual to you. What may be grossly high for one program might be just right for yours. In pricing programs, I look at what I have in the program and look at what I have bought and sold before that is similar. Then I pick a price that I feel is fair but will cause the clients to reach and commit and make this their number one priority for a short ninety-day period of time so they will absolutely get the results they are wanting and won't be distracted by life. Then I over-deliver. I continually look to reward my clients' investment and decision in me by finding more ways to add value in the program and go above and beyond and do what is required to actually get the result (not throw extra fluff that distracts but actual fine tuning, next level stuff that will deliver their absolute best results). When you set up an exchange this way, your clients feel great because they are committed, and they are getting results and they love it and you have raving fans. You are handsomely rewarded for what you give in your program that makes you want to show up even more and assist them in any way you can to get amazing results. So now both parties—you and your client—are connected and focused in the same positive direction on the map. You are moving onward and upward!

This is then sustainable and nourishing to you. You can sleep again at night. These fans of yours now can give you testimonials that lead to more ideal clients and a regular filled practice. This is the best way to scale organically. So, start with even one client. Serve them to your absolute best ability and for a price that feels good to you.

If you are extremely new, you could do a few free sessions to hone your skill and increase your confidence, but *you* will be getting the results not them. So, if you truly want to assist *them*, charge a price that feels good to you. Then with your next few clients increase your price as you add more value to your program. Your clients will have questions or situations that arise and when you answer them, you will be creating a continually better program for future clients, so price accordingly.

In Chapter 5, we talked about creating a signature program that is scalable. Initially one-to-one is fine (great actually because you really understand where your clients are coming from and how best to serve them). But there is a limit to your income here that may or may not be consistent with your goals. We played with some numbers in that chapter and realized that if you charged $1,000 for your six-month program, you would max out at about $60,000 with fifteen clients per week which is actually a very full practice that may or may not be sustainable. Even if you doubled that price to $2000 that is still not likely to reach your goals in a way that is sustainable. From Chapter 3 when we focused on "What did you want—what did you really, really want?" There was a vision for what you wanted to do with your program and how much you wanted to earn. What were those annual and monthly income numbers? What was the vision you had? Do you want to get to the point where you retire from your previous career? How much do you require to get there? If you have other streams of income from yourself or a partner, you may be able to allow this to grow gradually and you may be able to quit your day job earlier to fully pursue your dreams with your signature program. Or if you currently are not personally earning an income and this income is a bonus, you can also gradually allow this to build and scale. But still—allow it to build and scale continually. If you aren't growing, you're dying. You will want time for your family. You will want time for vacations. You will want time for you. You will want time. So, incorporate a leveraged component that we discussed in Chapter 5 so that it is scalable.

But what about if you are the sole or primary income earner as I was and both—your medical career and your developing coaching career—take a lot of your time? What if you are paid extremely well in your medical career and there just isn't enough runway to give you enough time to get your coaching career off the ground at a level that it matches your medical income so you can make a smooth transition to a coaching career and live happily ever after? It just isn't going to happen. Which is why what I did—to the outside observer—seems like a magic trick. So here is the inside scoop. First you really need to follow all of the steps I have been outlining in the *Awakening Process*. They are *all* important. There is no fluff.

Let's get real. You require a real program that delivers real results in a real way to real people that really want it and will pay real money for it. The simple steps that I have outlined in this book after a decade of experience and trial and error are the massive shortcut to this. Next as you start to serve your clients, you want to ensure you have a leveraged component of income, so you don't run out of runway before you have lift off. I love online courses and group video calls for this. You still deliver excellent world-class content, but it gives you more time. Next see if there are ways you can start to "downsize your life." As I shared in Chapter 1, I loved my dream home but not more than me and I couldn't sustain it as I tried to create this coaching career. This doesn't mean worse—just different focus. It requires a mature mindset to really trim your discretionary spending.

It requires you to focus on those things that are really important to you and those that you are willing to forgo for now. To become a doctor there was great personal sacrifice of your time, money and youth, and putting up with short-term pain for long-term gain. For your freedom and to fully satisfy your calling and enjoy life again, are there things that you are willing to sacrifice?

The things I did to downsize to create time and money to build and live into my dream included downsizing our home twice. The homes were always beautiful, and we made them all better than when we bought them, and I love to decorate so this wasn't necessarily a bad thing. We went without family or personal vacations (other than for business) for six years. We moved to a beautiful town that we didn't really want to leave anyways—so again this wasn't necessarily a bad thing. I gradually cut back on my medical hours by changing locations (and flying to work) to an excellent Calgary clinic where I no longer had on call responsibilities. This gave me more time to increase my coaching practice. There were a couple of income opportunities that also came my way that were in integrity with my beliefs and assisted me in serving my clients in an even greater way that helped to bridge the gap as I phased out my medical career and built my coaching career. I spoke as often as I could at wellness events or for corporations. I coached as much as I could. I learned from others—from audios, videos, books, conferences, podcasts, coaches, and mentors as much as I possibly could. I did not watch television for at least six years. There was just no time as I was navigating both my medical career and my growing coaching practice. This also made it easier to keep a positive focus so again it wasn't all bad. We did enjoy occasional movies. I rarely bought clothes—just what we needed with no shopping sprees of my previous life. Our clothes were just what we required, and we appreciated them and made them last. Fortunately, I still had clothes from my earlier days, and I had invested in many great staple pieces that stood the test of time, and my four boys and husband were at one point a perfect hand-me-down ladder for one another. Now they are all about the same size and particular in their style once again—so prior timing was great. We gave up going to any restaurants at all for about four to six years. Again, that allowed for better nutrition at home, so it wasn't all bad. I no longer had excess income to buy my sons many things they wanted (like I had when I was working as a full-time radiologist), but they learned to appreciate what they had and take care of it.

My husband who had sacrificed his career to stay home and raise our boys when I was a full-time radiologist had now been out of the work force for a long time and was still needed at home with our school age boys as I flew away to work in these transition years. He renovated and landscaped and maintained our homes, helped me with the tech and admin of my business, and we continually re-evaluated our rapidly changing situation and roles. I became aware of where I was investing my time, money, and focus. I couldn't be sloppy with any of those three. I invested in programs, education and mentors that would hasten my dream come true. I took those baby steps with consistent positive focus in the direction of my point "B" Bliss, and resisted (as best I could) the temptation to judge it too soon as not working. The map and elevator tools and everything I have shared here were the key ingredients that were the secret to my success. I made these short-term sacrifices (with no guarantee of success much like I did when I flew to spend twelve hours a day in the hospital with my dad for the six weeks of his stroke) and it was so worth it!

I have shared the raw truth you may not want to have heard. But the awesomeness is also absolutely true. If I had not have left my hospital position, I probably would not be here. I thought about suicide a lot in those days. I just couldn't see any way out. It was not sustainable. If I had not have left my medical career, I would not have fully fulfilled my calling to serve and truly heal. I would not have learned how very much the body is the miracle that can heal itself if we give it half a chance. I would not have learned that we have a choice and our choices do matter. I would not have learned that we can achieve the impossible. I would not have helped thousands of people with weight loss. I would not have been there for my children in their adolescent and teenage years. I would not now be happily married to my husband for over twenty-five years. I would not have been able to drop everything to be with my dad and witness and be a part of a medical miracle. I would not get to walk my dog every day through the gorgeous woods with my husband in my most favorite city in the world, Kelowna. I would not have been able to wake up when I am done sleeping. I would not have been able to drop everything and fly with my mom to celebrate her eightieth birthday in Hawaii, and travel to have a party for her in Winnipeg. I would not be able to tuck my kids in every night—even though they are now in their teens and twenties. I would not have been able to speak to thousands in Miami as the emcee and speaker of a two-day event for Joshua Rosenthal's Institute for Integrative Nutrition where Deepak Chopra was the keynote. (And yes, I got to chat with him backstage and hold the curtain open for him.) Being on stage with these two visionary men, who a decade ago I had stumbled upon during my late-night desperate web search, felt like the most delicious full circle moment! I would not have been able to help other health coaches who were just like me—with a burning desire to heal and make a difference but saw no possible way to do this—create their very own signature programs. I would not have made the difference I truly wanted to make. So yes, this was so worth it! I earned my freedom and you can too! If I can do it so can you! I am nourished now at a very high level. My clients are nourished at a very high level. Our souls are satisfied and eager for more. You can do this!

Now with consistent income from your world-class signature program, you will fully step into the leader you are becoming! In the next chapter we are going to talk about growing yourself and growing your movement! It just keeps getting better and better from here!

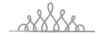

Chapter 11

Grow Yourself; Grow Your Movement

"Everyone wants to live on top of the mountain, but all the happiness and growth occurs while you're climbing it."
–Andy Rooney

What I have discovered is that success is not something that you get but rather it is something that you live into and become each and every day. A key component of creating and launching a successful signature program that transforms and makes a difference is becoming that person who is at the top of your mountain leading your tribe. It is an identity shift. The person that you are at the beginning of this journey as you start to create your signature program with your doubts and debts is not the same person as the leader of a signature program of a thriving movement that is making a difference. If you are the same person as you are at the beginning, doing the same things, eating the same things, hanging around with the same people, you are going to be making the same income and making the same impact as you are now. When you walk your clients through your program you are walking them through a transformation from point A to point B. As I help health coaches to create their own signature programs, I walk them simultaneously through their personal journey from point A to point B where they are the leader of their movement serving their tribe.

But as we become that new person we are going to bump into resistance. Part of us wants to stay where it is familiar. We actually need to kill off an old part of us with old habits and beliefs that are not serving us and step into a new way of life with new healthy habits and beliefs that are aligned with our new best version of ourselves. But we don't really like getting rid of our old familiar selves no matter how much it is haunting us and holding us back and sabotaging us every step of the way. People often refer to this breakthrough as busting through their comfort zone to get to where they want to be. I like to refer to this as your familiar zone. Because we are always going to want to do what we can to stay comfortable. That is natural. But most confuse comfortable with familiar and they are really uncomfortable in their familiar "comfort" zone. It is what they know. As you attempt to leave a familiar elevator floor of Guilt, Shame, Doubt, Disappointment, or Frustration, it can be hard to get past everyone and everything saying "Don't leave us. This is where you belong. You know everyone here." But you can't get to your point B—your desired destination of bliss and freedom and joy—from there. Not ever.

People want the point B results, but they don't want to change themselves or get in the elevator and go up to the *Neutral* lobby and *Satisfaction* mezzanine and hop in the *Love* elevator. They want the doctor income and credibility without going to medical school. They want the man of their dreams without doing the work to be the woman that attracts that man. They want a thriving six- or seven-figure coaching business without doing the personal work to become the owner of a six- or seven-figure coaching business. So, when you leave something familiar to try something new it can feel a little awkward. When you try a new haircut, try a new sport or skill, it can be awkward. My friend David T.S. Wood says, "Every master was once a disaster." This is true. It is going to feel weird to step into something new. I used to take private figure skating lessons before school and loved doing jumps and spins, but you can bet the first time I was on skates, it was awkward. When you start a new job, it is a little scary as you step into a new role. But have you ever done something where you just took that eight seconds of courage and just showed up anyway and walked into the room as if you were the person that you wanted to be? If you have never tried it, I encourage you to do it. Watch how others respond to you differently when you show up differently. When you stand up tall, head held high feeling and looking confident in your own skin, people respond to "that" person.

I remember once reading something you can try: think of someone you admire. Think of someone who you admire for their look and style and "wear" them. Try them on like a coat. I remember Sophia Loren was one of the examples they used. Try walking and talking and carrying yourself as if you were that "character." Adorn yourself with the essence of who they are. *Your* version of that. Or maybe it is a blend of characters. What would they do? How would they act? You see that over and over with the same "character roles" played out throughout history with slightly different nuances. Consider Marilyn Monroe, Madonna, and Lady Gaga. They *became* the person they are today. They literally adopted a new identity including a name change. You don't have to change your name but own and become the new best version of who you are—of who *you* want to be. I saw Lady Gaga interviewed after she starred in the movie *A Star Is Born* where she played the character Ally with her original brunette hair and minimal to no makeup, unlike the person we know as Lady Gaga. The interviewer told her it was really cool to see the "real" her on screen. To which the actress, with her signature platinum blonde hair and dramatic eyeliner, replied pointing to herself "This is the real me. This is who I really am. Ally is a character." The way she looks and acts *is* who she is. It is who she has become. It is who she is comfortable being in her own skin. None of us gets to judge for another who they should be or want to be. If we consider ourselves stripped of all of our accessories as the only version of who we are, then I suppose you could say homeless people are the most accurate representation of who we really are. But that just doesn't seem right. I don't believe that circumstance dictates who we are. Who we truly are is pure wellness. How that looks for each of us will be different. These accessories such as our speech, mannerisms, personality, clothes, hair can be an extension of who we truly are. You get to choose and as always, our choices do matter. You can literally choose to become the person that you want to become. You can choose to *be* the leader of your movement—first—before even the movement.

Something I teach my clients is to identify their attractive archetype. So, consider the ideal client you want to attract. Consider the leader that you want to show up as for them. If you are going fishing, you want to have the right bait. There are apparently over seventy archetypes and I first started to study this after listening to Deepak Chopra talk about how stories of characters, in the form of gods and goddesses in Greek and Roman mythology, in history, in soap operas and in modern leaders, were similar stories and themes carried out repeatedly. Others have stated that there are twelve primary archetypes that provide a foundation for your personality, beliefs, motivations and actions. These can assist you to strengthen your brand identity to reflect the hopes and dreams of your clients and attract them. Your attractive archetype sharpens your identity, so you are quickly identifiable. The twelve primary archetypes are:

1. The Innocent
2. The Hero
3. The Regular Guy
4. The Nurturer
5. The Creator
6. The Explorer
7. The Rebel
8. The Lover
9. The Magician
10. The Ruler
11. The Jester
12. The Sage

We see these roles and characters played out all of the time in movies (and in life) and these characters are instantly familiar and recognizable and thus, attractive to us. They are instinctive. They are part of our collective unconscious. As Carl Jung states, *"There exists a second psychic system of a collective, universal, and impersonal nature that is identical in all individuals."*

Each of these archetypes embody a core desire and fear and can be great or not in their extremes. There is no right or wrong answer. But some will lend themselves more to some people and some topics than others. The innocent archetype embodies simplicity and is great for childhood brands. The explorer archetype embodies freedom and is great for outdoor adventure and nature-seeking brands. The rebel on the other hand is leading a revolution and rejects the status quo and is great for movements that lead an alternative to mainstream doctrine. The lover embodies passion and glamour and is great for chocolate or luxury or relationship brands. The jester is all about fun and entertainment and a very playful brand. The sage is all about wisdom and more information with higher learning and vocabulary and would be great in university and hospital settings. I teach this in more detail to my clients in my course, but the purpose is to bring awareness to effective ways to optimally show up for your clients and to lead your cause. You have a choice and you can be intentional and strategic with it. This brings clarity and alignment between you and your movement and your clients. Progress then moves swiftly as you get to enjoy playing your role as you carry out your soul's purpose. This is much like I felt as I flew to be with my dad when he had his stroke. It was almost like I took on a persona of nurturer and hero that allowed me to be stronger than I could have been if I had just played the role of daughter seeing her dying father. I never accepted that role. I chose rescue hero—rooting for the underdog as I always do. Eternal optimist. Passionate nurturer with a dash of sage. Having that MD behind my name helped to take on that "role." If I had just been the daughter, I probably would have crumbled. I have done this too when results weren't as optimal as with my dad. The results aren't the important point here in what I am saying, but rather the strength you draw in becoming the best possible version of yourself at the moment. Have you ever had to rise to the occasion? Have you ever had to almost become someone else to succeed? Well you can do that on purpose in advance.

Everything that I have just shared with you here is the mystery ingredient as to why some succeed, and others fail when all else is equal. This is an important accelerator in your success and in fact makes the difference between having a six or seven figure business and never launching at all. This is a massive shortcut. Throughout this book we have alternated between the mindset and mechanics to create and launch a successful heart-centered business. Both are important. As you plod along through the mechanics you will gradually adopt an improved mindset. However, a fun hack is to adopt the mindset first. Become that person first. Then watch as all the details just fall into place with greater ease and flow with the right people showing up to assist you as you scale your business to the next level. Because if you are that person, you do things that enable (not disable) your success. This helps you ride the Love elevator to the Belief floor. This helps to protect you from your former you.

As I coached people, I realized how important this piece was to create real sustainable results and prevent self-sabotage. I could help someone lose 100 pounds, but in order for these results to be sustainable we had to address "who they really are" and how they saw themselves. If someone loses 100 pounds but still sees themselves as someone with an obese identity, they will self-sabotage themselves to be in alignment with how they see themselves. So, you can create the mechanics of an amazing signature program but if you see yourself as confused, hesitant, and doubting in your ability—it won't work. The leader of your movement by definition is a leader. The person you are as the leader of a massively successful signature program and health coaching practice is different than the person who started out wondering who you could help, how you could help, and uncertain as to if this would really work.

How do you create the identity shift to create and sustain amazing results? Well, first it is going back to where all of this started in Chapter 3 when you created a vision of what you really wanted. Imagine living into your dream come true. You have the best signature program. You have your dream life and business set up. What does that look like? Where are you? Who are you with and what you doing? Now close your eyes and imagine the person living this dream life. Just like we created a character story of who your ideal client was in Chapter 4, now create a bio of the person that has created their signature program and is leading that movement and making the difference you want to make. Who do you want to be when you "grow up?" Grab a pen and write that down. Answer questions like:

- Where does she live?
- What type of work does she do?
- How much money does she earn?
- What is she known for?
- What does she look like?
- What does she wear?
- What does she eat?
- What does she do? What does she not do?
- What does she say? What does she not say?

- What mannerisms does she have? How does she carry herself?
- What are her character traits?
- Which archetypes most align with her?
- How does it feel to be this person?

Keep writing any details that you want as you visualize this person (your future self) gliding through her day. Really consider what does this person do? She is probably not playing games on Facebook. She is probably not complaining or whining. She is probably not wasting time. She has probably learned to get out of her own way. Seek expert counsel as required. Accept assistance where warranted. She probably accepts 100 percent responsibility for the floors she is choosing and does not let others push her buttons...or if they do, she does not step out onto that floor for any length of time. This little exercise will help to bring your success character into sharper focus. Feel free to create a vision board that captures the essence of this person and the lifestyle that is truly your dream come true...because you are creating it.

As you keep inching forward with baby steps to create your signature program and launch and scale it and grow your movement, bring yourself along with you. Grow you. This is not about being someone who is fake or being someone you don't want to be. This is about moving more quickly into the best next iteration of yourself and not staying stuck. Because as you become the holistic entrepreneur, the master coach, the health professional leader you were born to be, your world-class program will be the natural extension of you. As that person, anything less just won't do. Self-sabotage is not an option. That is for those still stuck in the F elevator.

One final tip: Owning your power statement from Chapter 6 helps you to show up as that person. Professional photos do as well. Many of my clients literally up-level themselves when they get professional photos. They start to show up as the person in the photos. Just like a doctor shows up when the white coat or the surgical scrubs go on, your photos can help to strengthen your identity as the person you are choosing to show up as. Give your clients your best self. They deserve that. Be queen or king of your mountain! As you show up as your authentic aligned soul-satisfying self you will be naturally attractive.

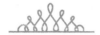

Chapter 12

Challenges Putting Theory into Practice

"In theory there is no difference between theory and practice. In practice there is."

–Yogi Berra

S tatistics show that most people never actually read the books they buy and especially not past the first chapter. So, if you are here—congratulations! That says something about you *and* me. You already have demonstrated focus and discipline and a winning desire. Throughout this book as you have journeyed through the *Awakening Process*, there were many practical steps and exercises to do. We continually blended the mindset and mechanics required to build a successful signature program. But just like your clients know they should eat more vegetables, actually doing it is another story. Having both the mechanics and mindset are an excellent head start but I thought I would fill you in on some of the potential pitfalls you may run into as you put this into practice and give you some perspective on staying true to you and your heart's desire.

As you know, all choices have consequences. We always have a choice (even if it doesn't seem like it because it is a rare choice). I remember when I was contemplating the choice to build a coaching practice after already investing my time, money and life into a medical career where I was now at the top of my game professionally but was feeling like the life had been sucked out of me. I couldn't see how I could last much longer. Do I do this crazy thing and start over in my forties? Will we survive if I leave? Will I survive if I stay? The lyrics to the song by The Clash kept going through my head: "Should I stay or should I go now? If I go, there will be trouble. And if I stay it will be double. So, come on and let me know. Should I stay or should I go?" This question was all-consuming. I thought about it every waking minute. All along I had been receiving nudges and wake-up calls to follow my true calling—my soul's purpose—that I shared in Chapter 1, but still it was a hard decision. I don't know what the right decision for you is. I do know there is more than one right answer. I do know from experience that following my soul's purpose was, as my friend David T.S. Wood described the process of launching a business, "Hard at first. Messy in the middle and gorgeous at the end!" For me, it was so worth it! But at the beginning I did not know that at all, and it was definitely not smooth sailing all the way. It took me at least $100,000 and a decade to fully transition over...and it didn't have to be that way! I probably made every mistake you can make along the way—giving too much for free, making it about me, talking too much, trying to heal everyone, doubting myself, hiring the wrong people, not hiring the right people soon enough, and especially just holding myself back not realizing it didn't actually have to be hard. Like fumbling around in a dark room, trying to make it light without actually touching the light switch. Just turn the lights on! Just flip the switch! Especially if someone you know and trust has been there and is pointing right to the light switch.

This is the biggest impetus for me to write this book. I know how painful that stuck indecisive limbo land is—not wanting to let go of the paycheck—not being able to tolerate the work much longer— not knowing if you can really make it on your own—especially when most people don't succeed in a sea of unsubstantiated hype—not knowing what to do. So that is the purpose of this book but let's take a look at you and your options and what you want because only you know your situation and what you really, really want.

First doing nothing is an option. Maintaining the status quo and staying where you are may be a great option for you. The Map and Elevator tools may be great mindset tools that totally change your perspective. Your current career may be the soul-satisfying work that you have always dreamed of and you have plenty of freedom. Then great (Although you probably would not be with me here in this chapter if that was the case)! But if you have a great plan A that is working for you—do that! Not everyone has a toxic work environment or feels stifled in their ability to make the difference they were born to make. Be good for you!

If your current situation is not working for you and you want to break free and truly make a greater difference healing, then consider what your options are costing you and how you can make the best of them. At the hospital and with my developing coaching practice it was obvious to me the killer effects of insidious stress. We sort of can be numb to stress because as we look around at the hospital, everyone else is doing it and at the moment they are still standing so…it is tempting to believe we can probably get away with it a little longer… until you can't. I saw several health professionals die on the battlefield of cancers, heart attacks, suicides every year. I saw many more suffer through painful divorce. I saw many more gain more and more weight. I saw many more become bitter, jaded—mere shells of their former selves. I am hard pressed to recall any health professionals back then that were the epitome of "health and happiness." So how about you? Where are you in the trapped in stress versus living in freedom spectrum? What is staying put (which is totally an option) costing (or benefitting) you?

Of course, leaving and creating your signature program is not necessarily a walk in the park either. It can be—eventually. It can be totally worth it. But if where you are is really great it might just be best to stay put because the path of the holistic entrepreneur is not without its obstacles which is why it took me nearly a decade to totally break free. However, that was needless suffering for me and the people I served or rather waited to serve until I had my act together. This book is designed to bypass all of that and lay out the exact mindset and mechanics to break free with your own signature program after weeks and months, not years and decades. But there are five main pitfalls that I want you to be aware of as you venture out and create your program, so you can avoid them with greater ease:

1. *There is a general culture of negativity that surrounds most of us.* Look around and notice how often people including yourself are tempted to focus on the obvious aspect of what is not working rather than what is working. Much of my time with my (truly positive) clients is spent redirecting and

reframing their assessment of situations to focus on what is actually working and what they do like. Hardly anyone does this consistently, but it often goes unnoticed unless I call it out. This is after years of focus on this for me and I still catch myself slipping into frustration or overwhelm. It is extremely helpful to surround yourself with a supportive culture of positivity that does believe in you and that lifts you up rather than holds you back.

2. *Not knowing what you actually want.* This is surprisingly more common than you might imagine. People usually know what they don't want. So, when asked what they want, the answer is often "Not this!" which is a great starting place. However, if we want to set our GPS on our map to our desired destination, we need to know what that is. It seems like it should be obvious but often we don't dare to dream that good or that big. We believe in the impossibility of improvement and can't see a way out. That is exactly where I was when I shared that story in Chapter 1 of a pager (that sounded just like mine) going off during a meditation on the question "What do I want?" at a Deepak Chopra event. That question had me stumped until that pager went off. I didn't think it was possible for me as a doctor to *not* be on call for the rest of my life but that is actually what I really wanted. Paying attention to clues, journaling and working it through with a coach or mentor can help to refine your focus further so you have a clear target to reach.

3. *Not knowing what baby steps to take.* In Chapter 6 we talked about the importance of inching forward with baby steps and I shared specific beginning baby steps. You took the step

to get crystal clear on what you do and create your power statement and then use that to test your offer. That is a very powerful and fun step. My recent group of health coaches as they went through this step had great results. One health coach today just posted that she received a great referral from a doctor following the *Awakening Process* and her client practically begged to be accepted by her. Another coach in the past couple of weeks had two new clients and last week seven more. Another was asked to create a six-week program in the community. These coaches knew the baby steps to take and refined it. It was a lot of fun to celebrate with them in the group knowing that they are making a great difference already and they are only a few weeks into the program. But perhaps more importantly are those where there isn't a client coming right away. Then what? What is the baby step to take then? Well we focus on the elevator. Assess the floor they are choosing. Focus on what is working and refine to make it work better. We look at whether the language is in the form of an eight-year-old. Are they talking about one specific problem or did they slip into trying to help everyone? Are they trying to take too many steps at once? Are they discouraged because they are not at six figures yet when the goal is just to have a conversation with prospective clients? Should the next step be to further narrow the niche or switch niches altogether? After all the purpose of the beta offer is to test it and see. Fail forward. But it is nice to amplify your chance of success and shorten your costly learning curve by knowing the next steps to take. Baby steps in the wrong direction are not helpful. Here is a simple example. Most of my clients have long distance phone plans and they call me, but I have unlimited long distance so if my client does not have it, I will call them. So recently I called one of my clients at her scheduled appointment time and there was no answer. That was unusual. I checked my calendar for the time and number and dialed her again. Still nothing. I looked into her previous spot on my calendar for her number. Dialed. Still nothing. Double checked my calendar software for her number (which I had filled out myself after her previous appointment) and dialed again. Fifteen minutes later she called me wondering if our appointment was still on. It turns out I had two digits flipped in her number and it was written that same incorrect way in all the places that I had transferred it from the original place of error. It didn't matter how many baby steps I took. I was not going to get my desired outcome if these steps were in the wrong direction.

4. *Inability to see your own blind spots.* This is common because we don't know what we don't know. This most often comes up in the area of picking a niche and owning your expert status in an area. We may have solved the problem easily or have been living in the solution for so long we forget that it is a serious problem that people are looking to solve. Those are some of the best niches because you have mastered it, but it may be so well mastered that you discount its value. I see blind spots with my weight-loss clients as well. I had a client with a hormonal medical condition who was really quite impeccable with her eating, but she had stubborn weight and bloating for twenty years that would not go. As she explained what she ate in detail, there really wasn't

anything obvious so we were going to go to the next level of investigation before ascribing it to her condition (which can virtually always be overcome because who we are is pure wellness—a topic for another book perhaps). As we probed further it turns out about twenty years ago, she fell in love with balsamic vinegar. She had it every day several times a day on her salads. When we did an elimination diet for seven days, her bloating vanished. Now I am not saying there is anything wrong with balsamic vinegar. I eat it on occasion. It does have sulfites and some people are very sensitive to that. And it may even be related to her medical condition. However, there was improvement when that was eliminated. She may not have to avoid it entirely (because she really loves it) but now she knows that it can trigger bloating in her and she gets to decide how she wants to be good for her. The point is that she never mentioned balsamic vinegar in a food diary because it was like nothing. No calories. Something she did every day for twenty years. It was like not mentioning you put ice in water. We all have blind spots and often when discovered these can bring swift changes.

5. *No one believes in you.* This is probably the biggest obstacle because if you are firmly planted in the Love elevator and you are on the Belief floor, you are golden! You got it! But if no one else around you has seen anyone else create a signature wellness program and make a living and a difference with it and live happily ever after, they are going to think you're nuts! They can't understand why you can't just stay in your day job like everyone else. They don't understand why you just can't be satisfied with where you are or what you have. They don't

understand why you are walking over to the elevator and keep pushing the button to go up and move up to a better floor. They don't even know there are better floors. People for generations may have lived on the same floor and they can't understand your burning desire for more and to satisfy your soul. That doesn't even make sense to them. What is a soul anyways? The more you try and explain how you feel and what you want and why—the more you realize they can't hear you unless you go out of the elevator onto their floor. Having a confidante and someone who is like-minded to brainstorm with is extremely valuable. This is why there are mentors and mastermind groups. The right group can have a powerful effect to lift you up and cause you to expect and believe more. My mother has been a great general confidante and she is my go-to person most often but in those early days in her loving way to protect me from the journey I was about to embark upon, she naturally had her own doubts and fears about it as did my husband, and neither of them are in the health or coaching worlds. So, investing in the right coaching and mentorships and high-value groups has been invaluable. Although investing in groups that are on lower floors than you or not aligned with what you *really* want can actually inhibit your success. When it comes right down to it there were absolutely days when no one believed in me, but me—and even then…I remember taking note of that—because if I ever got out of my soul sucking life alive, I was going to tell people who would dream of following in my footsteps that this was important to know and one of the hardest things to gut through alone. That is why in my

Awakened Healers group, the one thing that these coaches get in avalanches from me is belief. I don't accept just anyone in my program, however. I hand pick the talent that I know has the goods to succeed. So, then I can, with complete integrity, breathe that belief right into them. I give them all of the mechanics, all of the mindset tools, all of the tweaks and I love them up, praise them up, and show them the way to who they really are. These powerful loving leaders who are fully capable of leading their cause and making this world a better place is who they really are. I am right there in the trenches pointing out what they can do—what is working. I have video testimonials from some of my clients in the program at DrShaunna.com site and on my *Dr Shaunna* YouTube channel that you are welcome to watch if this is something that interests you.

Of course, what I tell everyone all day every day is "Be Good For You!" Everyone's situation is unique. Focus on what you really want. Consider what are the consequences to you and your family if you stay where you are and don't create a thriving health coaching career and what if you do decide to create your own signature program. Consider and beware of some of the pitfalls I have outlined here. But also, what are some things you can do to make your chosen path easier, faster, more fun and more of a sure thing? You can do this—if you want to—and it can be fun.

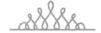

Conclusion

"Those doing soul work, who want the searing truth more than solace or applause know each other right away."
–Rumi

This book was written in response to the many questions I received over the years, as health professionals saw that I had actually broken away from my medical career to fulfill my soul's purpose to truly heal and make a difference. From their perspective, as I said at the beginning, it seemed like some sort of magic trick. But in reality, it was actually a repeatable specific process that could be duplicated. Although it took a huge investment of time and money to come to the conclusions that I have shared in this book, it did not have to be that way. But I didn't know of anyone else who had done what I wanted to do. There were no footsteps or roadmap to follow. But recalling my breakthrough journey in response to your many questions and inspired by the miraculous outcome of my dad where my process was clarified, put to the test and confirmed, I created a framework—a roadmap—The *Awakening Process*—should anyone want to follow in my footsteps to do their version of this "magic trick."

You now know this *Awakening Process*. Each step is important. Beginning with *Awakening to your soul's purpose* so that you are climbing the right mountain and building the business and life that *you really want*. Anyone can create a business or a program but if it is not what you really want, you will struggle. You want to define your destination on your map. Then it is important to know *Who you want to and can serve*. Keeping that specific ideal client in mind is key to your success and helps you come from love. Then you want to *Align your signature program to be the best solution* to solve your client's specific problem in the best possible way, allowing you to become world class. Then you just *Keep inching forward with baby steps*. Create your power statement and test your offer with a beta program and ensure you are on track and refine accordingly. It is important to keep positive focus in the forward direction and *Elevate yourself to your soul's purpose*. The elevator tool I developed is extremely useful for myself and my clients. I use it every day, all day to be aware of what floor I am choosing and prevent myself from falling into the basement where many people remain trapped for a lifetime. Then as you assemble the mechanics of your program you *Name the steps in your signature program* that walk your client from their specific problem to the specific solution. All along the way it is important to be aware and *Identify your influencers*. It is a lot easier to be massively successful when you are surrounded by positive influencers rather than negative ones that may be sabotaging you without you realizing it. For not only your success but your client's success, it is important to *Nurture your clients and yourself.* Being comfortable with receiving as well as giving and appreciating the transformative role that the loving exchange of money embodies is an important and often missing link for healers. Finally, to truly break free and live satisfyingly into your soul's purpose, you want to *Grow yourself and grow your movement.* Done right, there is no limit to the joy, freedom, abundance and difference that you will create from this process.

I appreciate that some of this can be easier said than done which is why I also shared some of the pitfalls that you may encounter as you go to put this into practice. Even if you have struggled before and still feel doubt, you are not the same person that picked up this book. You know more than you did at the beginning. You now know the mechanics and the mindset to succeed in creating your soul-satisfying signature wellness program that allows you to make a difference and a living.

The key components I want to re-emphasize here are to get crystal clear on what you want, awaken to your life's purpose and then take the baby steps to get there. Continually find ways to increase your positive influencers and avoid the negative. This really is one of the most important things. Finding a like-minded community is very powerful. In medical school, the other medical students were a like-minded community that made it easier. But also, the fastest path to success in anything is to find someone who has what you want and do what they did. This is why my prior four- and five-figure investments in mentors always paid off. But it still took me longer because I didn't know of another doctor or even another health professional who left a lucrative medical career to create a thriving soul-satisfying signature program that would still support her family at a very comfortable level. So that is why I am sharing this with you. If I can do it, you can, too! But the details do matter which is why I was very open in outlining the mindset and the mechanics.

This *Awakening Process* is something that I now teach to my clients to bring structure, steps, timeline, support, and accountability to nebulous dreams to make them come true. My clients may enter the *Awakened Healers* program somewhat confused and uncertain, but they emerge with clarity and purpose with their very own signature program knowing exactly who they serve, how to attract their ideal clients and how they can deliver the best outcomes. It is important to put all of this into practice as we go, and it is common for coaches to attract clients in the first half of the program as it is being created which is great practice for them to fund their movement as they grow. This is so important because your healing work is more important than ever!

You don't have to look very far to see the sad state of health in the world and especially North America. Over seventy percent of adults are overweight with nearly thirty-eight percent obese! Childhood obesity has tripled in the last generation. Adult obesity has quadrupled since 1986. The World Health Organization states that chronic complications of weight kill 3.4 million adults annually! Excess weight shortens life expectancy by three to fourteen years. Someone has a heart attack every thirty-four seconds in the United States. One in three women and one in two men will get cancer! Autism has increased from one in 10,000 children in 1970 to one in sixty-eight currently! Alzheimer's is now the sixth leading cause of death! Fifty million Americans have autoimmune disease! I used to say seventy percent of this could be prevented with a healthy lifestyle, but I feel like it is more like ninety percent since even in the past twenty years we have gone rapidly in the wrong direction! The world needs *you!* The world needs you *now!* People are literally dying for your help! This is the reason I broke free to do this work. To fulfill my calling to truly heal. But I alone cannot do this. To witness, many talented, loving, heart-centered health professionals with a burning desire to heal, but unable to do so because they are trapped in jobs that are sucking the life right out of them or they just can't figure out how to make this work is heart-breaking and needless. The world needs your healing work. You need to connect to the world that needs your healing work too. I could not stand by and watch this descend any further. Now is the time for health coaches to rise. People can't do this on their own. They aren't. Medicine and hospitals definitely have their place, but they are not the place for this proactive lifestyle medicine to be effective. Your time is now to break free and make a difference and a living with your own signature program. Awaken your inner healer! Create your soul-satisfying program! Massively increase your impact, income and freedom as a master health coach and break *Free to Heal!*

Acknowledgments

I have wanted to write books since I was ten years old and the neighbor boy Joseph declared in my kitchen that he was going to be an author someday (and he is). My life, however, led me to medicine and to follow my calling to heal. But as an avid reader, I appreciated the healing power of words. But beyond a strong desire, this book would not have been possible if it weren't for the support and guidance of many amazing people along the way. It truly takes a village.

First, I want to acknowledge my maternal grandmother who joyfully encouraged me to "go to the head of the class" and whose death when I was fourteen launched my mission to help people live their longest, healthiest, happiest lives.

My life would almost certainly be very different or even now nonexistent were it not for Joshua Rosenthal—an incredible visionary and founder of the Institute for Integrative Nutrition and another visionary, world renowned author and spiritual guru, Deepak Chopra—who taught me to meditate and inspired my love of mind-body medicine. A late-night desperate web search led me to both of these incredible iconic men whose lights shone so bright that I could find them in my darkness. I learned so much from both of them and their programs. My work is heavily infused with their influence. They will never truly know the profound impact they have had upon my life and the subsequent lives of my clients. I am eternally grateful.

To my many health coaching clients over the past eleven years that helped me become a better coach and who believed in me and allowed me to serve them to the best of my ability at the time and allowed me to be a pioneer in growing a thriving health coaching practice. It has been an extreme honor.

To the medical doctors, who referred their patients to me to coach, who were forward thinking enough to recognize the value of nutrition and lifestyle transformation in overall health and to give their patients an opportunity to improve their health "on their own" with me. Thank you for your belief and trust.

To the life-changing work of Abraham, Esther and Jerry Hicks, whose teachings have been profound and enlightening and have inspired my consistent daily meditation and appreciation practice and have positively influenced all areas of my life. I want to also acknowledge the work of many inspirational authors and leaders—too numerous to count but including Wayne Dyer, Louise Hay, and Oprah Winfrey.

Of course, this book would not have been nearly as impactful, practical or even possible were it not for those initial Awakened Healers who allowed me to lead them to create their own signature wellness programs so they can shine their light and make the world a healthier, happier place in their own soul-satisfying way. I can't believe how quickly this amazing group assembled in under a week!

It felt like divine timing was at play. Thank you and I love you Nicole Hume, Jennifer Bago, Lana Kirtley, Tim Pedersen, Rachel Borntrager, Valerie McInnes, Jill Saunders, Dr. Catherine Straus, and Alex Lukey!

To Dr. Angela Lauria: Words simply cannot express my immense gratitude. Your mentorship and guidance were world class and absolutely instrumental in producing this book that has already made a significant difference in the lives of health professionals so they could get their healing message out into the world. Thank you, Angela—you are a true inspiration and leader! Thank you to Cheyenne Giesecke, Ramses Rodriguez, my developmental editor Ora North, managerial editor Moriah Howell, and the many others who worked behind the scenes to make this book possible.

To the Morgan James Publishing team: Special thanks to David Hancock, CEO & Founder for believing in me and my message. To my Author Relations Manager, Margo Toulouse, thanks for making the process seamless and easy. Many more thanks to everyone else, but especially Jim Howard, Bethany Marshall, and Nickcole Watkins.

I want to acknowledge my social media following, particularly my Facebook friends, who have been so incredibly supportive of this entire endeavor right from its inception. You are awesome. Your immense support truly has meant a lot to me.

Of course, I want to acknowledge my amazing family, extended family, and friends who have been so supportive of me throughout this journey and all my crazy endeavors. Specifically, thank you to my husband Gerald and four sons, Ryan, Matthew, Jordan, and Brennan, and my parents Joe and Val Bachalo. They are certainly used to me taking the road less travelled but my strong desire to follow my bliss and do the right thing, even if it is unconventional can be challenging for anyone in my vicinity that wants to be "normal" or "average."

Those words never really have been in my vocabulary. Thank you for your patience and understanding as I follow my soul's calling to help people to live their longest, healthiest, happiest lives.

Ultimately, despite a long history of denying my calling and myself, and feeling trapped in my soul-sucking life, I want to acknowledge me, for taking a stand, following my heart and trusting my gut, to serve in the best way that I knew, even if I had not seen it done that way before. To commit to then pass on everything I had learned "the hard way" so that others can now benefit much more easily if they too desire to break *Free to Heal* in their most delicious, soul-satisfying way, is the best gift I can possibly think of to give!

We are all in this together. If it were not for you, my treasured reader, these words and the value they contain, would not continue to be passed along and perpetuate the healthy exponential ripple. Thank you for picking up this book and being willing to explore the *Awakening Process* and to "Be Good For You!"

Thank You

Thanks for reading *Free to Heal*!

This isn't the end, but potentially the beginning of a major, exciting pivot point in your life!

Definitely put into practice the steps and utilize the tools this book has provided as you launch your signature program as a vehicle to create your own soul-satisfying dream come true! But I *love* results and I would love to help you out even further!

I'd love to hear more about your mission and the signature program and movement you would like to create! Contact me at https://DrShaunna.com or comment at https://www.facebook.com/TheHealthProfessionalAcademy/

Free Referral Letter to Work with Doctors:
Your business thrives on clients. Often the best referral source for your signature program are doctors. Please visit www.DrShaunna.com/health-coaches/ to download a free referral letter that you can

use to partner with your doctor so they can refer health coaching clients to you and your signature program.

Free Video Class:

You are going to absolutely *love* this bonus video training I did on "How to Make Six Figures with Your Signature Program" at www.DrShaunna.com/health-coaches/. In this training I did for my coaching clients, I break down the numbers so you can cast the vision for yourself of not only what is possible but what is probable and what is required to make it happen and some of the pitfalls to avoid.

Apply for a Free Strategy Session:

Do you have a burning desire to make a difference and a living with your own signature program and want my feedback? Fill out the application form at www.DrShaunna.com/apply/. It is my pleasure to connect with like-minded holistic entrepreneurs because when you are doing the soul-satisfying work you were meant to do, everyone wins!

Be Good For You!

Dr. Shaunna

About the Author

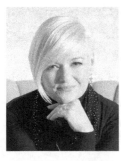

Dr. Shaunna Menard has been a medical doctor for over twenty-five years and is a Canadian and American board-certified radiologist. She is an international speaker and trainer, certified holistic health coach, superfoods author, former Chair of Public Health and former assistant professor of medicine, and she has spoken to international audiences of thousands on health and wellness, and has been featured on Breakfast Television. She is a visiting teacher at the Institute for Integrative Nutrition and has shared the stage with mind-body medicine expert Deepak Chopra.

Her grandmother's death when she was fourteen, galvanized her mission to help people live their longest, healthiest, happiest lives and led her to medical school. However, as a doctor, she observed that the majority of diseases could have been prevented with a healthy lifestyle. She knew within the medical system, it was difficult to help patients adopt the healthy habits that would lead to a significant, sustainable improvement in their health. She became frustrated with the rising epidemics of obesity, cancer, and diabetes. She worked extremely hard to get to the top of her career professionally but found herself unsatisfied and not truly fulfilling her mission to help people live their longest, healthiest, happiest lives.

She then made the bold, unprecedented move from the end of the line to the front lines to transition from burned out doctor to blissed out health coach. She works as a lifestyle medicine specialist at DrShaunna.com and has created a superfood meal planning service at MealCure.com. Her success leaving a lucrative medical career to create a soul-satisfying and thriving health coaching practice led many health coaches to reach out to her for advice. Observing the growing health crisis and the struggle and defeat of many holistic entrepreneurs, her mission expanded to inspire and empower health coaches to grow their business and heal the world and she founded The Health Professional Academy. She created the *Awakening Process*™ to teach health coaches how to create their own soul-satisfying signature programs that make a difference so they can enjoy greater income, impact, and freedom! Dr. Shaunna lives with her husband Gerald and their four sons and golden retriever Duke in beautiful Kelowna, BC, Canada.

Website: DrShaunna.com

Email: shaunna@drshaunna.com

Facebook: https://www.facebook.com/shaunna.menard

Facebook Group: https://www.facebook.com/groups/BGOOD4U/

YouTube: Dr Shaunna https://www.youtube.com/user/4Drmom